Praise for

BUILT TO SURVIVE: HIV Wellness Guide

Built to Survive is a key resource for anybody providing care for HIV patients. It is informative, innovative and accurate. I refer to it very often and recommend it to many of my patients and students.

— **Professor Julian Gold, MD**, Sydney, Australia

***

An excellent book full of good, sound advice that individuals can follow to help decrease some of the side effects of HIV/AIDS. A book for the individual, but also a highly recommended book for all medical, academic, and public libraries.

— ***AIDS Book Review Journal***, University of Illinois at Chicago

***

This book provides user friendly information about an extremely important topic, combined with a sophisticated and accurate presentation of the scientific evidence available to support the clinical recommendations.

— **Judith Rabkin, PhD**, Columbia University, New York City

***

Built to Survive provides an accessible overview of certain important therapies, by advocates who have made themselves experts in this area. We suggest this book as a source of ideas that you may later want to discuss with your physician.

— **John James**, *AIDS Treatment News*

***

Mooney and Vergel's most vigorous message is don't just depend on medicines to manage your health. Diet, exercise, and hormones, if appropriate, could help you achieve the healthiest body and strongest immune system possible.

— **Charlie Smigelsky, RD,** Editor, *Nutrition for Healthy Living*, Tufts University, Boston

***

See additional endorsements of this book in the Forewords and on the back cover.

BUILT TO SURVIVE
HIV Wellness Guide

Michael Mooney and Nelson Vergel

Forewords by
Mauro Di Pasquale, M.D.
Patricia D. Salvato, M.D.
Shannon Schrader, M.D.

HOHM PRESS
Prescott, Arizona

Cover design: Kim Johansen

Cover Photo by Matt Soileau, Houston, Texas

Cover Model: Aaron Molitor. Aaron is an HIV (+) man who had lost weight and was dying. He is healthy now, and is the personal trainer of co-author Nelson Vergel, who was also dying and had lost weight to 140 pounds. See Nelson's picture on the last page of this book.

Layout and design: Tori Bushert

Library of Congress Cataloging in Publication Data:

Mooney, Michael, 1953-
  Built to survive : the HIV wellness guide / Michael Mooney and Nelson Vergel;
forewords by Mauro Di Pasquale, Patricia D. Salvato, Shannon Schrader.– 4th ed.
    p. cm.
  Includes bibliographical references and index.
  ISBN 1-890772-43-7 (pbk.: alk. paper)
1. AIDS (Disease)–Hormone therapy. 2. Anabolic steroids–Therapeutic use. 3. Weight loss–Prevention. 4. AIDS (Disease)–Patients–Health and hygiene. I. Vergel, Nelson, 1959- II. Title.
    RC606.6.M66 2004
    616.97'92061–dc22

                          2004020671

HOHM PRESS
P.O. Box 2501
Prescott, AZ 86302
800-381-2700
http://www.hohmpress.com

This book was printed in the U.S.A. on acid-free paper using soy ink.
08 07 06 05 04   5 4 3 2 1

Formerly published as *Built to Survive: A Comprehensive Guide to The Medical Use of Anabolic Therapies, Nutrition, Supplementation and Exercise for HIV (+) Men and Women* by Michael Mooney and Nelson Vergel; Houston, Texas: Program for Wellness Restoration (PoWeR), Third Edition, 2003, ISBN: 0-9662231-0-1.

Our Vision

Until there is a cure, we envision a day when wasting and lipodystrophy syndromes will have clear, practical, and comprehensive standard of care guidelines with prophylaxis and intervention therapies that are cost effective and accessible to every HIV(+) man, woman, and child in the U.S. and around the world.

Disclaimer

The information contained in this publication is for educational purposes only, and is in no way a substitute for the advice of a qualified medical doctor, registered dietitian, certified nutritionist, or exercise physiologist. When you ask any professional to help you make your decisions about your personal healthcare, we recommend that you show them the information in this book, because they may not be aware of it and the scientific studies that support our recommendations. Appropriate medical therapy and the use of pharmaceutical compounds like anabolic steroids should be tailored for the individual, as no two individuals are alike. We do not recommend self-medicating with any compound, as you should consult with a qualified medical doctor who can determine your individual situation. Any use of the information presented in this publication for personal medical therapy is done strictly at your own risk and no responsibility is implied or intended on the part of the contributing writers or the publisher.

Acknowledgements

To those who have helped our efforts to carry this message.

In Memory of:
Michael Dullnig, M.D., for sparking this effort. His memory lives in this book.
Barry Chadsey, M.D., for having the guts to pioneer this therapy. Preston Keith, who helped Nelson find this life-saving therapy. My friend Richard Wiederholt, who was the wise man in Nelson's life. Alberto Lopez, for putting others ahead of himself. Chester Meyers, Ph.D., for his contributions to progressive nutrition for HIV. And to all those who have died from wasting syndrome. May God rest their souls.

Special Thanks from Nelson Vergel to:
Mauro Di Pasquale, M.D., for generously sharing his knowledge and bringing Michael Mooney into my life. Patricia Salvato, M.D., for believing in me from the beginning, even when most doctors were skeptical. My doctor Shannon Schrader, M.D., for his compassion, support, and selfless commitment to the HIV community. Gary Bucher, M.D., for initiating his groundbreaking anabolic study. Al Benson, for being committed to spreading the word. My life partner, Tim Baker, whose love and support has brought stability into my life that has enabled me to do this work without worries. My mother, Hilda, a woman who taught me the joy of helping others, and to my brothers and sisters, who have always stood next to me. Anthony Bianchi and Pete Sharpe, who believed in me and helped me create the Body Positive Wellness Center. Ellen Hahn, for being such a super-empowered, tireless and reliable volunteer. Jeff Taylor, for being a great supporter, friend and advocate for people with HIV. Roddy Grabert, my loving friend, who spent hours editing my work. Kathy Mulligan, Ph.D., for her great research mind and deep interest in what is good for the community. Our PoWeR advisory board members, for believing in this work. All progressive physicians, registered dietitians, nutritionists, and exercise trainers who help people by trusting their intuition before controlled data are available.

Special Thanks from Michael Mooney to:
My friend and research associate Jim Brockman, for sharing his intelligence and his insight. I could not have done what I have without his help. Mauro Di Pasquale, M.D., for introducing me to Nelson. Walter Jekot, M.D, for going against the grain. Al Benson, for his personal courage. Ellen Hahn, for her selfless

giving and for reminding me to have fun. Lark Lands, Ph.D., for her willingness to lead, where others follow. Fred Sattler, M.D., for accepting us as equals. The late Dan Duchaine, for his good advice and support. To Bill Phillips and T.C. Luoma, for delivering our message to 300,000 *Muscle Media* readers. To my mother, who has always been there for those who are less fortunate. To my sister Kathy and my father Patrick. If they had not let me have time away from work and given me their support, I would not have been able to do any of this. And for all the people who have benefited from our work and shared it with others, God bless each of you. We do this for you.

Contents

Foreword

by Mauro Di Pasquale, M.D.
Ontario, Canada

I was both honored and pleased that Michael and Nelson asked me to do a Foreword for their new book. This book has been a long time coming and is eagerly awaited by everyone who has been involved in fighting the devastating effects of the HIV virus.

I was fortunate enough to have known and helped the late Dr. Michael Dullnig, also known as "Dr. X" in *Muscle Media* magazine, in his efforts to spread the word about the devastating effects of weight loss in HIV and the often lifesaving effects of anabolic steroids. I corresponded with Dr. Dullnig back in 1993, and, after sending him my various publications, I advised and collaborated with him until his death in June of 1994. He was an intelligent, knowledgeable, and dedicated man, who made a significant difference in all of our lives.

Before his death, Dr. Dullnig passed the torch to Nelson Vergel. I remember when Nelson called me asking for my help, saying that Dullnig had sent him over a quarter ton of research material. From the first time I spoke with Nelson I had no doubt that he would succeed in his efforts to understand and apply the healing principles that would eventually make such a big difference in the lives of all HIV(+) men and women.

A short time after Dullnig died, I received a call from Michael Mooney, who was independently researching the use of anabolic steroids and other growth factors in AIDS. Realizing that they had so much in common, I gave Nelson's phone number to Michael in the hope that they would collaborate. On looking back, my giving Nelson's phone number to Michael was one of those meant-to-be kinds of things. The results of their collaboration turned out to be more than I had hoped for.

I have watched over the years as both Michael and Nelson have changed from being innocent idealists to being veterans in researching, speaking and writing on various aspects of HIV disease and its treatment. This evolutionary process has resulted in an astounding transformation, so much so that while at first I had much to teach them, they now have surpassed my knowledge and expertise on several fronts. Today, they are two of the most knowledgeable and dedicated people I know, and equally important, the most caring and unselfish. Without these special attributes, their work and this book would never have been. Together Michael and Nelson have made a difference to every HIV(+) person. This book is a culmination of their knowledge, hopes, and desires to help their fellows.

Michael and Nelson tell me that I am one of their role models because of my work back to the late seventies on anabolic steroids and other growth-inducing compounds, as well as my ongoing work on nutrition and ergogenic supplements. I am proud to have played a part in their accomplishments, but I am especially proud that they say they learned a lot about the value of substantiating what they say with references to the medical literature from my work. In our interactions over a number of years, I have encouraged each of them to go where others fear to tread, but stand on solid ground, and I think this book does exactly that.

Among many other things, you will learn how the judicious use of anabolic compounds, along with optimal nutrition, exercise and other treatment modalities, will increase longevity and dramatically improve the quality of life for those who are HIV positive. But while this book will help people with HIV learn about some important survival tools, that is not all you will get from reading it. This book, while important for its educational content and clinical information, is a testimony to what can be done against adversity and ignorance. What emanates from this book is the courage, dedication, and vision of its authors. For them, this book is but one steppingstone in their journey. One that will not end until a cure is found.

Foreword

by Patricia D. Salvato, M.D.
Houston, Texas

This book, by its very name, is reflective of survival – survival of the fittest. Michael Mooney and Nelson Vergel endeavor to shift the mindset of HIV as a terminal wasting illness, into a mindset of health-enhancing behaviors that can contribute to long-term survival. Even though there is no cure yet in HIV disease, a life of quality and value can be sustained in this disease. Continuing education for the physician has been a fundamental precept of the profession since the case descriptions of Hippocrates were used to understand prognosis. Physicians have always been expected to follow a personal plan for progressive learning throughout their practicing careers. The principles supported by Michael Mooney and Nelson Vergel have undoubtedly added to the full picture of care for my HIV patients, and have been an incredible learning experience in my practice.

This book reflects an encouraging public trend toward the assumption of personal responsibility for treating HIV disease. It urges the patient to take an active role in treating his or her condition, in combination with traditional medical treatment. The concepts in this book help strengthen the HIV patient's will to live, against the constant threats of HIV's desire to kill. I have seen in my practice that using all options and enlisting the patient's innate ability to heal has helped lead to long-term survivors. Drawing on my experience and that of the many exceptional people I have encountered and the many exceptional things that they have taught me has added a new dimension to the quality of life of my patients with HIV disease.

In HIV disease, weight loss has been associated with an increased risk of mortality in a number of studies, and also with an increased risk of hospitalization and in the development and progression of the disease. Regardless of T-cell count, body cell mass correlates with quality of life. Early studies noted a disproportionate loss of body cell mass compared to fat mass, and that depletion of body cell mass may start early in the illness, even before significant immune dysfunction is present. Studies have shown that as little as a 5 percent weight loss can increase morbidity and increase risk of infection. Anabolic steroids are receiving increased attention as a treatment, both for wasting syndrome and to prevent loss of crucial lean body mass. Anabolic steroids increase the retention of nitrogen in the body and promote weight gain and increased body cell mass, especially when combined with an exercise program.

Anabolic steroids are certainly no cure for AIDS, and their use, like all drugs, can produce side effects. However, the benefits far outweigh the risks, as side effects can all be easily managed with the guidance of a physician. Testosterone and anabolic steroids can provide the following positive effects:

Stimulate appetite

Promote muscle anabolism, reduce catabolism

Improve overall sense of well-being

Increase muscle protein synthesis

Stimulate growth hormone (GH) and insulin-like growth factor-1

Stimulate the immune response

By finding medications that reverse the depletion of body cell mass, we may be able to add years to the lives of our HIV/AIDS patients. I believe that we can increase the quality of life, and positively alter the CD4 T-helper and the CD8 suppressor cell counts and ratios in patients by using anabolic steroid therapy.

As we slowly approach a cure for this disease, anabolic steroids may be the missing ingredient necessary to prevent the body's premature depletion of its mass and thus prevent the descending spiral into life-threatening metabolic, endocrinological, and infectious complications.

The results of following the principles set forth in this book give HIV(+) people, for the first time, the power of self-esteem in this disease. Researchers are now studying the very strong relationship between attitudinal healing and immune function. I have learned over my years of practice that one cannot understand disease unless one understands the person who has the disease, and also the feelings of helplessness that the disease can sometimes create in them. We must all confront the reality that no one lives forever. Illness and death are not signs of failure; what is failure is not choosing to live. The goal should be to live with dignity and quality of life, making each day meaningful and life sustaining.

As I have watched my patients battle this disease, I know how courageous they are and how much they have learned about healing. I see in survivors how they embrace life, not how they avoid death. Those who learn to take the challenge of their illness and share responsibility for their treatment have chosen a path that leads to peace of mind and healing on both a spiritual and physical basis.

No two people manage their illnesses exactly the same way, even if they have the same disease, the same doctors, and the same treatments available to them. In the end, each person must manage his or her life in a way that makes sense to themselves.

This book represents much of what has been learned through collective experiences about HIV wasting syndrome and how to treat it, as well as about preventing the wasting that can accompany HIV disease. More specifically, it represents the fact that an independent will to live, combined with health-enhancing behaviors, can contribute to prolonged survival; even when cure is not possible, a life of quality and value can be sustained until the end. This book also teaches the patient to be informed and assertive, and not be shy about telling his or her doctor about this program and the successes that have been seen. Patients deserve the best possible understanding of their problems and the best treatment combinations. Combining knowledge from this book with the guidance of the medical profession will certainly enhance health, and lead to a long and more fulfilling life. *Built to Survive* should be helpful, not only to interested patients, but also to physicians and other healthcare providers dealing in the daily battle against HIV disease.

The comprehensive scope and treatment of this subject, the obvious expertise of the authors, and the interesting anecdotes related by a patient, present valuable information in an interesting way. But, this book also serves as a true foundation for patients willing to fight the fight, and for physicians facing the demands of HIV disease that require immense flexibility, tolerance, and an ability to have a true physician/patient relationship.

Foreword

by Shannon Schrader, M.D.
Houston, Texas

It is with great pride that I am able to contribute to this important book. Nelson and Michael deserve the highest amount of respect for venturing forward on what is still a controversial topic.

The advent of highly active antiretroviral therapy (HAART) in the treatment of HIV has significantly improved the survival for a person with HIV. In addition to HAART, other key components must be included in treatment in order to enhance this continuity of life. These essential factors include proper nutrition and exercise, additional nutritional supplements (e.g., vitamins, minerals, and protein), and frequently, the introduction of anabolic steroids.

Over the last few years, I have begun utilizing anabolic steroids in my private practice as an adjunct to HIV therapy. I can attest to incredible transformations that have occurred with the use of anabolic steroids. For example, I have witnessed reversal of the wasting syndrome –which has been virtually eliminated in my practice – improvement in libido, improvement of immune function, and stabilization of the physical changes associated with the lipodystrophy syndrome reportedly being manifested as a result of antiretroviral therapy. As people watch their bodies improve, they develop a more positive perspective. Even people who previously reported some signs and symptoms of depression speak of a better outlook on life. Improved mental health contributes to good physical health. A positive physical transformation empowers people to fight a little harder!

The greatest controversy over the use of anabolic steroids surrounds the issue of overuse. Abuse of anabolic steroids can cause harmful side effects, including, but not limited to, liver damage, stimulation of the prostate gland, aggressive behavior, depression, high blood pressure, and over-use syndromes of the joints. However, under the supervision of a physician knowledgeable in their use, anabolics offer many benefits for the person with HIV. One such advantage is the normalization of testosterone levels in men with HIV. Low testosterone levels are a frequent untoward effect of HIV infection. Hypogonadism (decreasing testosterone function) in HIV(+) people significantly correlates with the loss of lean body mass, decreasing T-cell count, and increasing morbidity. With maintenance doses of testosterone, hormone levels in the body can be normalized.

In addition to increased utilization of anabolic steroids in my practice, I am seeing continued incorporation of complementary medicine into Western medicine in HIV care. A holistic approach to HIV medicine is growing in importance. As a general rule, this approach is not taught in most medical school settings. However, I am learning on a daily basis from my patients that vitamin and mineral supplements are synergistic with standard Western medicine. Deleterious effects from routine HIV medications may also be treated with holistic remedies. I am witnessing marked improvement in the immune system and in the quality of life as a result of supplements.

Lastly, the benefits of proper nutrition and exercise must not be underestimated. These parameters are integral to maintaining a healthy immune system, and fundamental for living a healthy life.

My wish for anyone using this book as a guide is that he or she realizes how important each component is with respect to HIV care. The components – diet, nutritional supplements, exercise and anabolic steroids – are like pieces of a jigsaw puzzle. Each piece, in conjunction with antiretroviral therapy, fits together to maximize the treatment of HIV.

Michael and Nelson's courage and commitment, as required to follow through with the dream of publishing this book, are exemplary. Hopefully, for those who read and learn and grow from this book, their example will influence you not to give up, but to fight for life.

Introduction

This book details a comprehensive approach to reverse and prevent the critical loss of lean body mass called "wasting," while it also addresses lipodystrophy, the unusual redistribution of body fat that is being seen in many people who are taking HIV medication. It covers nutrition, supplementation, resistance exercise, androgenic-anabolic steroids, growth hormone, and other therapies. It is a compilation of the works of two people, each of whom bring different but complementary abilities to the table.

Nelson Vergel, a former chemical engineer, native of Venezuela, and long-term HIV(+) survivor, is a leading treatment advocate for HIV-related wasting, lipodystrophy syndrome, and wellness in HIV disease. In 1994, after watching friends die of wasting and facing wasting, Nelson pieced together a comprehensive program that allowed him to gain forty-five pounds of muscle and rebuild his own health. Determined to share what he had learned with others, Nelson created a non-profit organization called Program for Wellness Restoration (PoWeR), to help others learn how to rebuild their lives and their health.

Nelson's vision included the creation of non-profit wellness centers for HIV(+) people, educational tools, and research studies to validate the tools that comprise his comprehensive approach to wellness. During his three years as a community representative to the AIDS Clinical Trials Group, Nelson helped to move forward the agenda for more research into the treatment of wasting and lipodystrophy syndromes. Nelson has also written articles and been interviewed in numerous magazines on this subject.

In June of 1999, in Houston, Texas, over 100 volunteers from the HIV community helped Nelson open his first dream facility, the 4,000 square foot Body Positive Wellness Center. The Center contained a fully equipped gym staffed with certified trainers, nutritional evaluation by a dietitian, a dietary supplement buyer's club, massage/chiropractic therapy, stress management classes, and a conference room for wellness related seminars. The non-profit wellness center concept is devoted to helping HIV(+) people get healthy and stay alive until there is a cure. To say that his program has helped Nelson Vergel return to living with vitality seems almost an understatement when all is considered. He is his own testimonial to his work.

Michael Mooney, an HIV(–) nutrition industry insider, has researched holistic health since his early teens, and is a journalist. Far away in Los Angeles, because of efforts to help HIV(+) friends, Michael had independently discovered many of the same things about health related to HIV/AIDS that Nelson had discovered. After watching dozens of friends die from AIDS, and coming from a "family of activists," Michael found himself spending his spare time working as a volunteer treatment advocate, researching alternatives to the mainstream medical model and educating people about their treatment options. After Dr. Mauro Di Pasquale introduced them by telephone, Michael, ever the idealist, became Nelson's key support person and research partner as the Director of Research and Communications for PoWeR. Nelson's vision and Michael's knowledge joined forces.

Since their union, Michael has publicized their work by producing their newsletter and its comprehensive web site www.medibolics.com; been interviewed in *Sports Illustrated* as an authority on anabolic hormones; been quoted on ABC Televisions' *Good Morning America*; had articles published in numerous magazines and newsletters, including *POZ Magazine, Positively Aware, Ironman, Musclemag, European AIDS Treatment News, Provincetown Positive,* and *Peak Training Journal*; and for two years was a contributing editor to *Muscle Media*, where he became known as "the medical steroid guru."

Popular lecturers, Michael and Nelson lecture together and separately, and have collectively given over 400 presentations around the United States. Nelson has also given several lectures in Spanish in Latin America. Their abstracts or co-authored studies have been presented at the 1996 Vancouver International AIDS Conference, the International Conference on HIV and Nutrition in Cannes in 1997, the Geneva AIDS Conference in 1998, as well as other AIDS conferences. In addition, PoWeR co-sponsored the International Conference on AIDS Wasting in November 1997 that featured the world's leading experts on the subject.

This book is the sum of the information they have collected for HIV wellness.

Built To Survive begins with Nelson's personal story, because he is the quintessence of a person who is benefiting from this very progressive and very comprehensive approach. If you are suffering side effects like lipodystrophy cause by HIV medications, or your overall health has been severely compromised by HIV, this book will provide you with some of the most effective, easy-to-follow information about improving your general health, immune response, and lean body mass. It also gives you solidly documented information that will help you to convince your doctor to work with the progressive elements suggested here. This book will give you the tools. Now all you have to do is not give up. Keep your own hope alive and realize that until there is a cure, you can be healthy and strong while coexisting with this disease.

1
Nelson's Story
by Nelson Vergel, BsChE, MBA

I remember when I was eight years old and I asked my mother, "What is cancer?" She gave me the best explanation she could without alarming me, but I also remember saying: "If I ever get cancer when I am older, I am going to live life to the fullest, travel, and do something big before I die!" I do not know why I remember that, but maybe, it was self-prophesy. Later in life I ended up not getting cancer, but I found out I was HIV-positive in 1987 when I was twenty-eight years old. I was probably infected five years earlier in March 1982, when I first came to the U.S. from Venezuela. I met Calvin, the man who was to become my lover for six years on that trip. I went back to Venezuela and spent weeks with the worst flu of my life. Life went on as usual after that as I was unaware of what had started happening to my health.

Two years later, Calvin called to tell me that he could not wait any longer for me to move to the U.S. and, fearful of losing him, I sold everything, packed my bags and left my country. I had left years before when I went for school in Montreal, Canada, but now it was a true adventure. I moved to Houston from Venezuela in 1984 to start a new life with my lover, full of dreams for the future in the land of opportunity. After getting my MBA, I found good jobs in the oil and gas industry as a chemical engineer.

One day in 1987, Calvin came to me with the bad news that he had gotten tested for HIV and his results were positive. I realized that I had to be positive too. After crying for a whole night, I decided I had to face reality. I went to get tested. When the results came back, my counselor told me: "You are HIV-positive: go home and take care of yourself." Back then there was nothing to treat this illness, not even AZT. I realized that all my dreams were collapsing in front of my eyes. I had come to this country three years before with the idea that I was going to make it. Instead, I was now constantly thinking that an early death was going to rob me of my dreams. After grieving for days, I decided that if I was going to die, I would explore all possibilities first on how to stay healthy. I was extremely hungry for medical information. I subscribed to ten of the best AIDS newsletters in the country to keep myself updated. Additionally, a month after my diagnosis I enrolled in a training program with the Centers for Disease Control to become a certified HIV counselor, when the one who really needed counseling was me. Counseling more than twenty people a night gave me the strength to continue to empower myself. I became an avid reader and researcher about anything that had to do with AIDS and health. I was still working full-time as a chemical engineer back then, keeping this terrible stressor a secret from my employer and coworkers. No one noticed, and my job performance improved, probably due to my lack of fear about future expectations. I started a search for my real life purpose, something that would fill me with passion. I knew from several research studies on psycho-immunology that those with a life purpose tend to live longer. One thing I already knew – being a chemical engineer was not what I wanted on my obituary.

As time went by, I became more and more symptomatic. Diarrhea, anxiety attacks, thrush, skin problems, night sweats and other ailments became common struggles for me. I knew that I could not continue just doing what my doctors said, and that I needed to do something different if I wanted to stay alive. I enrolled in an AZT study, but realized that I was on a placebo (sugar pill) when my T cells kept dropping. I was also losing weight and energy. My relationship with my lover ended and I was transferred to Los Angeles from Houston in 1990.

I knew that there were more possibilities to learn about alternative therapies in Los Angeles. I was excited and scared at the same time, since I knew no one there. It took me awhile to get used to L.A. I started meeting people who were on the same search for health that I was. I got involved with very dynamic support groups where we discussed the latest treatments and alternative therapies. I started to consume mega doses of supplements, exercise regularly and to watch my diet for allergic reactions. My health started improving; however my weight was still decreasing. (I used to weigh 165 lbs. and I was down to 140 lbs.). I became more eclectic about my healthcare – I used the best that the pharmaceutical world and the holistic world had to offer. Many of my friends who were HIV-positive were against using antivirals, since they thought these heavy drugs weren't worth the side effects. I was fortunate to use them without any problems. I also realized that this virus is a very smart one. I came to the belief that switching therapies every six months or so would probably prevent a lot of the problems associated with viral resistance (mutations) and the side effects due to long-term use of antivirals. I am extremely

grateful about all that I learned while living in L.A. I consider that time the beginning of my transformation toward what I am today.

I got transferred back to Houston a year and a half later. I was a different person with a new perspective on my healthcare. I was more assertive so I demanded that my doctor let me take reasonable risks in my choices of therapies. In the mean while, Calvin, my ex-lover, and many of my friends were dying of AIDS. Most of them ended up looking like skeletons before their deaths. Calvin, a man who used to be handsome and well built, lost 100 pounds (from 180 lbs. down to 80 lbs.) and died in bones as we watched helplessly. I refused to accept that there was nothing the doctors could do to stop their wasting, which was probably the main contributor to my friends' deaths. I decided I was not going to be the next victim of my own and my doctors' ignorance in treating wasting. I became focused, and maybe obsessed, in finding an effective therapy to this dreadful illness.

One day in the summer of 1992, one of my friends in L.A. called to say that he had gone to a seminar about the use of anabolic steroids for AIDS. I remember saying, "But steroids are supposed to be bad for you!" I recalled all I had read about the abuse and misuse of anabolic steroids, about "roid rage," and about how you could get cancer and liver problems. My friends in L.A. insisted that the seminar speaker sounded like he knew what he was saying, and that this was probably a good option to reverse my weight loss and improve my quality of life. I was very skeptical, but in the back of my mind a little ray of hope started to shine. Maybe this was it!

I decided that I was going to do it. I figured that I had more to win than to lose. I tried finding a doctor who would prescribe the steroids, but could not find one. Friends of mine began trying to find dealers who could bring anabolics from Mexico. I also asked my mother in Venezuela to get me some testosterone cypionate and Deca Durabolin – they can be obtained over the counter there. I was finally able to obtain them and start this therapy, full of excitement, fear and hope. Months later I found out that Dr. Barry Chadsey and Dr. Walter Jekot in Los Angeles were already prescribing anabolic steroids to their patients.

I was very worried about the fact that I was doing something potentially risky without any guidance. I bought every bodybuilding magazine possible. They all criticized the use of anabolics and pushed their supplements as replacements. One magazine had an advertisement for Bill Phillips' *Anabolic Reference Guide*. I ordered it and was offered a subscription to Bill's magazine, *Muscle Media 2000*. I accepted it. It took me a few days to devour the book. I found it extremely helpful. However, I was still worried that there was nothing in it about the potential benefits or risks of anabolic steroid use on the immune system. I remember talking to my friends about trying to find a person who would know more about that matter. Hopefully, it would be a person who was HIV(+) and maybe a researcher or doctor.

My first issue of *Muscle Media* arrived and I read it hungrily. To my surprise and delight, there was an article in the magazine written by an HIV(+) doctor! This doctor, who called himself "Dr. X," had gotten out of his death bed, regained forty pounds, and gotten his life back by using anabolic steroids, even though he only had 4 T cells! I called my friends in L.A. immediately and told them that we had to get hold of this Dr. X. My friend Preston spent the next two days networking on the phone. He called me with the good news that he had found Dr. X's phone number.

I didn't hesitate to call Dr. X. He returned my call and we talked for an hour. His real name was Michael Dullnig, M.D. He was a psychiatrist on disability and was writing a book on his experiences, about his personal program. What a delightful, smart, passionate man. I became his number one

fan. We would talk for hours every week to share our experiences. I told him I was looking for a life purpose and that I was willing to volunteer some time to help him in any way to spread this information.

In the meanwhile, I gained good lean body mass. I put on thirty-five pounds during the next year or so. My immune response also improved, especially my CD8 T cells, which went from 900 to 2,500 cells per mm^3. My symptoms basically disappeared. I never felt or looked better in my life, even when I was HIV(–)! And all this happened before we even had protease inhibitors. I agreed with Dullnig that it was unethical and immoral to keep this information from HIV(+) people and doctors just because of all the misconceptions, stigma, and hype surrounding anabolic steroid use. I wanted everyone who needed this information to have access to it. None of the so-called information-based organizations out there had anything on anabolics and HIV disease, and only a few short papers had been written about it. Most doctors I talked to did not know much or anything at all, and some were very much against the use of anabolics because of all the bad publicity associated with them. So, I decided to embark on a crusade to gather more information and to help Dr. Dullnig to disseminate it.

Things kept getting better for me. My quality of life got to be the best I could remember; even my mind worked better. Unfortunately, that was not the case for Michael Dullnig. While I was fortunate to have started the program while my CD4 cells were still over 200 cells per mm^3, Michael started the anabolic steroids when his CD4 count had already dropped to 4 cells per mm^3 (normal range is 1000 to 1500 cells per mm^3). Even though he was able to live a good full year after he started steroids with his new quality of life, he eventually developed CMV retinitis (a viral infection that attacks the retina of the eye and makes people lose their sight). He called me to say that he could not stand the thought of going blind, and that he would rather die than go through the chemotherapy required to treat that infection. My first thought was to motivate him to go on, to finish his book. He called me weeks later to say that he had drawn the line and that he was going to end his life the next day on June 1, 1994. I was shocked. He was in a hurry to call everyone to say good-bye, so he did not have much time. He said that he was going to accept my offer to help him finish the book and spread this valuable information. He hung up and I spent hours crying in shock. A week later via Federal Express I got 650 pounds of research material that Dullnig had sent me. I knew my life was never going to be the same after that.

I started to get Dullnig's fan mail. I got dozens of letters, from all over, from people who desperately needed help. I realized how really important this work ahead of me was. I was still working for Shell Oil then, but could hardly concentrate on my work after that. It took me four months to digest all the information to be able to continue the work. I also did my own research by going to the medical library every week to read about nutrition, endocrinology, exercise physiology, and related fields. Since Dr. Dullnig had made me promise that I would not wait for the book to be published to spread the information, I decided to create my own nonprofit organization in Houston called PoWeR – Program for Wellness Restoration. I sold my house. I came out at work as an HIV(+) man, and told everyone about my new purpose in life. My boss was extremely supportive and told me to do whatever it took to find myself. I went on permanent disability at work in September 1994, and was able to devote myself entirely to my new project.

I created a workshop format with over a hundred slides and invited a few experts to join me. One by one they all came to me, seemingly effortlessly. Dr. Mauro Di Pasquale, a world expert on anabolics and sports medicine, was the first to join my efforts. Dr. Luke Bucci, author of several books on micronutrients in sports and recovery was soon to follow. Dr.

Lark Lands, one of the top nutritionists who specializes in HIV disease has also been a great supporter. Dr. Patricia Salvato, a very progressive and respected doctor in Houston, started using the program with her patients with great results. Then, life sent me another Michael to help me in this mission. Michael Mooney, a nutritional expert in Los Angeles who was also independently researching this field, called me after Dr. Di Pasquale gave him my phone number. Michael turned out to be a passionate, knowledgeable, and truly concerned individual who is committed to researching this area and to sharing this information with others. We became partners in this mission and he joined me in my travels around the country. In our efforts to share the information that we think is so important we have collaborated on this book and several other publications. Without him, my efforts would not be half as effective. Jim Brockman, another great mind, joined us later and added even more excellent research information to our work.

Because of our hard work, several hundred physicians and other healthcare professionals, including registered dietitians and certified nutritionists, are now endorsing and applying the program with thousands of HIV(+) people. Over a hundred HIV/AIDS agencies nationwide have used our services as seminar speakers. We have designed and implemented or been involved in the design of several research protocols to test our comprehensive program.

PoWeR is now a 501(c)(3) nonprofit organization. We have given our *Built to Survive* workshop in every major city in the United States, and many smaller U.S. cities too. I have given a presentation to the largest medical school in Venezuela. We presented our "Anabolic Hormone Guidelines" at the XI International AIDS Conference in Vancouver in July 1996, and at the XII International Conference on Nutrition and HIV in Cannes, France, in April 1997, and had a poster presentation at the XII

International AIDS Conference in Geneva in June 1997. We have been quoted in *AIDS Treatment News*, *POZ*, *Sports Illustrated*, *Positively Aware*, *MuscleMag* and *The Advocate*, as well as numerous newspapers and other publications, and been interviewed on several radio and television programs. We established our newsletter, called *Medibolics*, and its associated Internet website. We helped create the Houston Buyers Club, a nonprofit organization that sells supplements at a discount for HIV(+) individuals nationally through mail-order. With the help of 100 volunteers I created my dream facility, a one-of-a-kind one-stop Wellness Center in Houston with another agency, Body Positive, to provide free or subsidized supervised weight training, nutritional counseling, body composition analysis, chiropractic massage therapy, and other services to HIV(+) individuals with limited income. I have lobbied to include wellness services in the Ryan White federal funding system for Houston. PoWeR has an advisory board with very distinguished doctors and researchers who are experts in clinical applications and in research about wasting and nutritional medicine. I was asked to join the Wasting Committee at the AIDS Clinical Trails Group (ACTG) in Washington, the largest HIV/AIDS research organization in the world. We also cosponsored the first International Conference on AIDS Wasting in Fort Lauderdale in November, 1997, with 27 speakers and 178 participants. And, we have been able to do all this with no federal funding, and very limited educational grants. We feel that sometimes all it takes in life is fearless commitment. I truly believe that conviction, passion for what I believe in, and the love of all around me have kept me alive more than all the medicines I have taken. I also believe that HIV was not a "bad" coincidence in my life, but one that enriched me and made me live life to its fullest.

We still struggle to find funding and free publicity to be able to do this work, and have used lots of our personal money to spread this important message. We hope that as time goes by more and more people will realize how important this work is, especially now, in the era of the new protease inhibitors, when people are living longer and want to take better care of themselves. Wasting is not a thing of the past. Recent data shows that as many as 30 percent of HIV(+) people are still having problems with maintaining healthy lean body mass. A lot of people are experiencing an unusual redistribution of their body fat, a phenomena that is being called "lipodystrophy," while losing lean body mass. Wasting still has no standard of care. Funding for our kind of work is very limited and will only increase when people, corporations, and the government realize the importance of maximizing health and productivity in a population that was thought to have no future.

No matter what, I can honestly say that we will never give up. With communications from numerous HIV(+) people thanking us for helping them live with new vitality, Michael and I both find this to be the most rewarding experience of our lives.

After five years of work, we first published this book with funds we raised from our seminars. All author proceeds from the sale of this book will help fund HIV-wellness-related projects in the U.S. and other countries. This book is a great avenue for us to share with you what we've found in our search for more effective and healthy ways to enhance lean body mass, quality of life and productivity in this critical illness. It took five years of work, but I think the wait was well worth it. Peace and good health.

2
Jump Start Your Life with Anabolic PoWeR
by Nelson Vergel

Optimal nutrition, supplementation, exercise, rest/relaxation, and hormonal intervention have been demonstrated to be essential elements for increasing survival for many people with critical illnesses. Higher amounts of lean body mass, not fat mass, have been correlated to increased survival and slower disease progression in AIDS. But, how does someone go about obtaining the needed information to preserve or enhance lean body mass, immune response, and overall health?

People rarely find this information readily available through their physicians. Many doctors have not been properly educated about nutrition, the therapeutic value of exercise, or hormonal therapies. Regarding the potential medical uses, safety and efficacy of testosterone and anabolic steroids, they are misinformed by an educational system that has been compromised by politics.

A study performed by the American Society for Clinical Nutrition in 1991 showed that only 20 percent of medical schools required courses in nutrition, and only one school had an independent nutrition department. Additionally, nutritional advisors such as dietitians, who work with doctors, are generally very conservative about their recommendations, and do not know about the cutting-edge information regarding dietary supplements that often have the most positive effect on our health. Even so, most HIV medical practices do not even include a dietitian on their healthcare team.

Moreover, some medical doctors only prescribe problematic drugs approved for wasting by the FDA. Megace, for instance, was shown in one survey in 1996 to be the number one drug prescribed by over 90 percent of the HIV doctors in the U.S. Yet, Megace has been shown to increase mostly fat content, and cause high blood sugar, kidney problems, blood clots, and a decrease in testosterone production in men, which renders them impotent. It can also promote lipodystrophy, the unusual fat buildup and redistribution (associated with protease inhibitor use) that alters body shape. Only the most progressive doctors in some cities will prescribe drugs like anabolic steroids for an off-label use, or evaluate you to determine your nutritional status. So, it is left to the patients to save themselves by searching for the best resources in order to learn about nutrition and wellness.

Learning all there is to know about how to stay healthy can sometimes be overwhelming. It can even seem to be a full-time job. But, a lot of this information is common sense; things you may have heard from your grandmother. It took me years to gather information about wellness, nutrition, exercise, and mind/body control techniques. I wish someone had come to me back then with all the information I needed on a silver platter. If I can help it, I do not want other people to have to go through the long process that I went through.

Although I have probably been HIV(+) since 1983, it was not until 1994 that I started becoming very symptomatic, experiencing thrush, diarrhea, weight loss, sweats, hairy leukoplakia, and skin problems. I became desperate to regain control of my health. Doctors were able to treat my symptoms, but nothing was being done to stop the downward spiral in my health. I realized that only *I* could save myself from what seemed to be inevitable. I was also watching as many of my friends were wasting to death, and nothing was being done about it. I guess some caretakers used to assume, "Well, he's got AIDS, and that is the way AIDS patients are supposed to look and die." Well, I want to make this statement loud and clear: You do not have to waste away if you have AIDS! And, you do not have to feel frail, with low energy and no drive to live. I have found that there is a lot of new and old information now available to reverse and prevent wasting, and to improve overall health and well-being.

Listen to what ACT-UP has been saying for years: Ignorance = Death. The information in this book can be an antidote. Fortunately, after gathering this information and applying all that I have gathered, I am glad to say that most of the time I am basically healthy, feeling and looking the best I have in years. Although this program isn't a cure, it definitely has improved the quality of my life, no matter how many or how few years lie ahead. Yes, it takes a lot of dedication and requires lifestyle changes. But with patience and perseverance anyone can do it. Now that people with AIDS are living longer, it is more important to take care of ourselves. We can remain healthy until a cure for this epidemic has been found.

Let's review the main elements of what I think you should know about wasting, nutrition, supplementation, exercise, hormonal therapies, state of mind, and general wellness for HIV disease.

1. **Understand the myths and facts of nutrition in critical illness.**

   a. Eating more does not necessarily mean that you are going to gain lean body mass; only good quality foods will help you build a healthy body. Proper diet may also help reduce the potential for lipodystrophy. (See Chapter 12, *Complementary Approaches to Treating Lipodystrophy*.) Resistance exercise combined with proper nutrition is the key for enhancement of lean body mass.

   b. Taking a multivitamin that contains 100 percent of the Recommended Daily Allowance (RDA) does not mean your micronutrient needs are covered. Studies at the University of Miami School of Medicine determined that most HIV(+) people need six to twenty-five times the RDA of many vitamins, minerals, and antioxidants to reach cellular levels that are needed for overall health. Also, a study of 296 HIV(+) men, conducted by researchers at the University of California at Berkeley, showed that those taking vitamin supplements over a six-year period were 31 percent less likely to develop full-blown AIDS than those who did not. Nutrition is one of the most neglected frontiers in AIDS. Many HIV(+) people simply die from malnutrition.

   c. Fat is not a four-letter word. Many of us need more healthy fats in our diets for the health of our immune systems, optimal lean body mass growth, proper fat metabolism and vitamin and mineral absorption. Intake of specific healthy fats may reduce the potential for lipodystrophy, while intake of other fats can increase it. Also, low-fat diets can make it very difficult for you to gain lean body mass. *Read about proper dietary fat intake in Chapter 20, Orthomolecular Nutrition.*

d. Eating well does not mean less nutritional supplementation. Studies show that even HIV(–) people have a difficult time getting enough essential nutrients. HIV disease dramatically increases your requirements, no matter how many CD4 T cells you have.

e. Because the lean body mass supplies fuel to the immune system, lean body mass is critically important for long-term survival. Your total body weight is a good indicator, but knowing your body composition and lean body mass is a significant key to detecting early-stage wasting.

f. You may be losing lean body mass even though your body weight has not changed. In early wasting, fat and water content can be increasing at such a rate that you continue to weigh the same but are actually losing critical lean body mass. Body composition analysis via bioelectrical impedance analysis (BIA) should be a standard test that you are given when you are diagnosed, just as viral load and T-cell counts are.

g. Increased fuel needs, caused by fighting the infections that come with HIV, can be the main cause of weight loss when food intake and other factors cannot explain it.

h. Aerobic exercise can cause you to lose lean body mass, so it should only be done when you are healthy and your lean body mass is stable. It can also probably help those with increased abdominal fat that has been caused by lipodystrophy.

i. Nutritional education/intervention should be provided as soon as someone finds out that he or she is HIV(+), not when they are already wasting, which is generally in the middle and late stages of the disease.

2. Understand that you are in control of your healthcare decisions.

Physicians are trained to treat symptoms, and sometimes they may not be proactive enough to keep you healthy unless you are assertive (and even aggressive) about your own choices. You should become your doctor's partner in your healthcare, and not assume that he or she is going to take care of you without your own efforts. Physicians are very busy people who sometimes do not have the time to update themselves with the latest information. Educate yourself and bring any new information to your physician's attention. Ask a lot of questions. Some registered dietitians are similar to doctors in that their methodology is generally very conservative, so they usually won't suggest the more progressive nutritional techniques. While there is good reason for the conservative approach of the mainstream medical and nutritional people, the HIV community has benefited from many things that have not gone through the typical review or approval process. And HIV(+) people often do not have the luxury of waiting until something is proven to be effective. Finding new approaches that are effective *right now* can extend and improve our lives. Keep your mind open.

3. Be an empowered and well-informed consumer.

Keep good records of your blood work; demand copies of all lab tests and ask to be taught how to read them. HIV(+) people fuel a multibillion-dollar medical industry. A study in the February 1995 issue of *AIS Patient Care* found that the monthly estimated cost for care for the first six months after AIDS diagnosis was $2,764, and people with advanced AIDS were likely to spend $9,098 on monthly medical costs (before protease inhibitors). However, HIV medication costs can amount to more than $15,000 per year. Considering the expense, it is only fair that we get optimum healthcare. We have to demand sound pro-active care through nutritional intervention, among other avenues.

It has been many years since this disease was recognized, and we still are dealing with basics like lack of good nutritional advice for people living with HIV. Demand recommendations from your physician. He/she is obligated to refer you to a licensed nutritionist or dietitian covered under your insurance. Also, inform yourself by subscribing to newsletters such as *AIDS Treatment News* (415-255-0588), *Treatment Issues* (GMHC, 132 West 24th St, New York, New York 10011), *BETA* (800-327-9893), and *Critical Path AIDS Project* (215-545-2212). Subscribe to Internet newsgroups like "lipidlist" and the "PI treatment list." Study Chapter 20, *Orthomolecular Nutrition*, in this book. Also, read books like *Healing HIV* by Dr. Jon Kaiser. Information obtained from these sources will keep you current and also give you the tools to hold intelligent discussions with your healthcare practitioner about your treatment options.

4. Engage in optimal nutrition.

To compensate for the increased basal metabolic rate encountered in HIV that tends to deplete lean body mass, work to improve your nutritional intake, especially protein intake, which is key to building lean body mass. This is detailed in Chapter 20.

5. Ensure optimum supplementation to compensate for high oxidative stress in your illness.

Several studies have shown a strong correlation between taking supplements and extended lifespan. The rapid turnover of HIV, and the death of T cells on a daily basis, can cause increased catabolic cytokines (protein messengers in the immune system) and free-radical damage of cells. Several studies have investigated the use of antioxidants, carnitine, and B-vitamins to minimize the mitochondrial toxicity cause by HIV antiviral medications. (For our recommendations for daily nutrient supplementation, see Chapter 20.)

6. Find out what your nutritional status is.

Most people take supplements and eat a good diet but still do not know whether or not their requirements are being met. As I said before, highly oxidative stress is typical of critical illnesses like HIV disease and cancer, but we are all biochemically different. The recommendations presented above are good starting points, but readjustment of dosages of micronutrients are needed after your nutritional status is determined. There are techniques currently used by many physicians to determine your micronutrient, and antioxidant status, to detect malabsorption problems, and to determine what foods or compounds create an allergic response that burdens your immune system. There are several tests that help to determine someone's cellular vitamin/antioxidant status, allergies, and gut absorption, including SpectraCell's "EMA" and "Spectrox" tests, Pantox's "Antioxidant Status Test," Sera-immune Physicians "Elisa/Act" allergen tests, Great Smokies "Digestive Analysis" tests, and body composition tests, among others. Consult a physician or dietitian.

7. Start a resistance weight-training exercise program.

The most efficient way to stimulate the body to increase lean body mass is through resistance weight training. Note that aerobics won't substitute for weights. Weight training has also been shown to improve people's quality of life and strength. Most of us are fatigued and do not think we can exercise. However, starting slowly and conservatively will get you started and help you adapt to this lifestyle change. (See Chapter 25, *Weight Lifting for Maximum Muscles Gains*, the weight-training section in this book, for the exercise phase best suited for your energy level and disease status.) Aerobic (cardiovascular) exercise is also important to decrease excess body fat, decrease elevated blood sugar and improve blood lipid profiles to reduce cardiovascular risk.

8. Get hormonal intervention (for those metabolically challenged).

Due to the high basal metabolic rate (BMR), catabolic cytokine activity, inadequate energy and caloric intake, hormonal disturbances, and other factors, some HIV(+) people need testosterone and anabolic steroids like nandrolone decanoate (Deca Durabolin), stanozolol (Winstrol), oxandrolone (Oxandrin), or oxymetholone (Anadrol). Anabolic steroids are synthetic analogs of the body's natural anabolic hormone testosterone. These compounds increase protein utilization for muscle growth (anabolism), increase appetite, stamina, libido, and help to produce a feeling of well-being. Although they are illegal for use for those with no justifiable medical condition, they are perfectly legal by prescription for people with wasting diseases. Many HIV specialists prescribe them on a weekly or semi-weekly maintenance schedule to prevent wasting, or in a ten- to sixteen-week high-dose cycling manner for those who have already lost over 10 percent of their body weight. Anabolic steroids do not help build optimal lean body mass without proper nutrition (specifically adequate protein intake and optimal calories) and weight training. Sitting at home watching TV will not make your lean body mass grow,

although rest is extremely important in any wellness program like this. (See the chapters on anabolic steroids [15-19] for more details)

9. Learn, Labor, Love, Laugh, Let Go.

Dr. Barrie Greiff, formerly a psychiatrist at the Harvard Business School, believes that a positive approach to life correlates with health and happiness. He suggests that certain personal habits are advantageous. His five L's of success are Learn, Labor, Love, Laugh, and Let go. Following these suggestions allows you to embrace life with involvement, challenge, empowerment, and fun.

Approach each day as a chance to *learn* (be open to new experiences); *labor* (at something that satisfies you and brings meaning to your life); *love* (give, recognize, and receive); *laugh* (with yourself and others); and *let go* (release things that are out of your control). If you feel alone in your battle, you should know that you are not. Thousands of people are going through the same awareness experience. Get out and meet them. Join support groups and organizations in your area. Most HIV/AIDS service organizations are hungry for people who want to help others. Get out of your shell and invite them into your life. Isolation is dangerous to your mind and to your survival.

3

What is AIDS-Related Wasting?
by Michael Mooney and Nelson Vergel

Wasting is defined as the involuntary loss of 10 percent or greater of normal body weight. It is specifically caused by the catabolism of lean body mass, which results in overall weight loss. The lean body mass includes the body cell mass, water and bone. Body cell mass is basically all the metabolically active cellular mass in the body. This includes muscles and organs (heart, lung, kidney, etc.), but not extracellular water and bone.

We do not agree with the Center for Disease Control's current definition of wasting. No data can be found on why this 10 percent definition was selected. Dr. Macallan of St. George's Hospital Medical School in London, has determined that 5 percent involuntary weight loss is enough to significantly increase risks of opportunistic infections (OIs). Also, no body composition data is included in the current definition. A revised definition that also includes losses in lean body mass (or body cell mass) and total weight loss of at least 5 percent should replace this obsolete definition, one that was created years ago in a time when there was little information about this syndrome.

When the body is fighting infection, and has urgent requirements for various biochemicals to deal with the tremendous metabolic stress it is confronted with, it requisitions many of these biochemical compounds from the body's most accessible storage area, the lean body mass. These tissues are metabolized (broken down into different components like amino acids, protein, sugar, fluid, lipids, etc.) to fuel the body's response to HIV and HIV-related diseases.

For our purpose, we will discuss the loss of lean body mass and the body's use of what it contains that fuels the immune system's defense against infection. It is important to note that there is not one single cause of wasting in HIV disease, and there are numerous possible agents that are involved in effecting the breakdown of lean body mass, including cytokines, neurotransmitters, prostaglandins, nutritional deficiencies, and hormones.

For simplicity's sake, the important consideration is that the subset of the lean body mass that is the muscle tissue is more than just tissue that functions to move the body. The muscle tissue is the primary reservoir of an amino acid called L-glutamine that is used to fuel the generation of the immune system's T cells.[1,2,3] T cells are cells that fight infections like HIV in the body. So the muscle tissue's role as a storage area for L-glutamine is absolutely critical to the immune system's effort to fight HIV and other infections.

When wasting begins to happen, usually after HIV disease has progressed to some extent, there is a progressive loss of lean tissue. This can take place as a series of events over many months. For instance, a person could have an infection, like any number of

HIV-related infections or even something as common as the flu. Each time the person experiences one of these events, the body takes L-glutamine and other metabolic fuels from the muscle tissue to support the immune system's response to the infection. This causes some loss of muscle mass. When the person gets well, he or she may regain total body weight, so that his weight as measured on the doctor's scale is the same as before he was sick. This can be deceptive, though, because typically in the earlier stages of HIV people don't regain as much lean tissue as they have lost, but they do regain fat and water to equal the amount of total body weight that they had before the illness. So it seems like their total body weight is normal and that everything is okay, but really, they've lost lean body mass and are in the early stages of wasting. Over the next several months, this same thing may happen a number of times. Each time the person loses a little more lean body mass, while regaining some fat and water. Eventually the progression accelerates and begins to bring the person's total body weight, including fat mass, down. At this time it becomes obvious that he or she is wasting, because the scale actually shows a loss of total body weight. It is unfortunate that the loss of lean body mass was not detected earlier, because it is easier to reverse wasting and stay healthy if it is detected in the early stages.

That is why we recommend that doctors calculate lean body mass using Bioelectrical Impedance Analysis (BIA) instead of the traditional weight scale, which only measures total weight. (See Chapter 6, *BIA and AIDS Survival.*) This type of analysis can give a fairly good relative reading of body cell mass versus total body weight that can be used to detect loss of lean body mass when it first begins to happen, usually before any weight loss registers on the bathroom scale.

Critically important is the fact that, after wasting has progressed beyond obvious weight loss, eventually there is not enough lean body mass to provide fuel for normal metabolic functions. As a result, the person dies. Dr. Donald Kotler showed that, on average, death occurs when lean body mass falls to 54 percent of normal.[4] Therefore, it is of utmost importance to stop the progress of wasting and reverse it as quickly as it is detected. Additionally, it is a good idea to gain additional lean body mass above what is considered to be average, as insurance against any quick loss caused by future infections. So, it may be advantageous for a person with HIV who normally is light-framed and thin to work to gain extra lean body mass.

While there are numerous drugs like protease inhibitors and antibiotics that are employed in dealing with HIV and the different infections that can accompany it, the accessible drugs that serve as truly effective and relatively benign wasting-therapies are limited to androgenic-anabolic steroids and growth hormone. Each is discussed in this book. There are several issues and misconceptions regarding wasting syndrome. The next chapter details some important ones.

For a better definition of wasting that was developed by Dr. Donald Kotler, Dr. Corklin Steinhart and Dr. Bruce Polsky, visit http://www.hivandhepatitis .com/hiv_and_aids/lipo/wasting/1guidelines.html. Print this page out and give your physician a copy.

4

Wasting Syndrome Treatment Issues
by Nelson Vergel

Wasting is among the greatest main killers of HIV(+) people in the U.S.

   (Source: Centers for Disease Control)

Wasting is among the top three main killers of HIV(+) people in the world.

(Source: World Health Organization, 1997)

- Two of the drugs that are most commonly prescribed for wasting are actually appetite stimulants. These drugs are Megace and Marinol. Neither of them is a true wasting therapy. Megace is a progesterone (female hormone) based compound, that effectively increases appetite, but studies show that it causes mostly fat gain, and can cause impotence in males, excessive menstrual bleeding in females, and hyperglycemia. Marinol is a synthetic derivative of marijuana, and it too is effective for increasing appetite, but without the kind of serious hormonal and metabolic side effects that Megace can produce.

- Some physicians wait until wasting is evident to start intervening. Prevention of wasting should be as important as prevention of opportunistic infections like pneumocystis carinii pneumonia (PCP). Monitoring body composition periodically with the use of BIA should be part of the standard of care in HIV disease. It is vital to detect any changes in lean tissue because, as Dr. Macallan has determined, just 5 percent unintentional weight loss is enough to increase the risk of opportunistic infections significantly.

- Many physicians think wasting is a thing of the past. As you will read in the upcoming chapters, people taking protease inhibitors are regaining mainly fat mass when they gain weight. The terms "protease belly," "truncal obesity," and "buffalo hump" are used to describe what is being observed in some people. Fat mass is being stored in the midsection and behind the neck, while muscle mass and fat is being lost in the extremities. Women with HIV have problems not only with truncal obesity but also with enlarged breasts. It seems that wasting is still present but it may be simply wearing another face.

- Human growth hormone (GH) is a drug that was approved for wasting, but its price and recommended dose make its use a luxury most people cannot afford, even if they are insured. While GH does have valuable fat-burning effects, a comparison of the studies conducted so far indicates that GH does not produce as much lean body mass gain as appropriate doses of nandrolone decanoate, testosterone, or other anabolic steroids. (See the comparison table on GH versus anabolic steroids in Chapter 18, pp. 77-88.) And while GH can increase lean body mass somewhat, it appears to have no effect on muscle growth for many HIV(+) people, as most of the lean body mass gained is simply water, not muscle. Significant muscle gain is accompanied by measurable gains in critical strength tests. Studies do not show GH improving critical strength tests.

- Much anecdotal and research information from HIV(+) people, progressive HIV physicians, and researchers points to the fact that anabolic steroids, an economical but politically stigmatized treatment, are highly effective in preventing and reversing wasting and improving quality of life for HIV(+) men, women, and children. It has taken years for controlled studies to be started due to the lack of interest from the pharmaceutical companies (patents expired in the 1960s for most of these compounds). Community-based trials are the primary potential source of the data needed to make this treatment approach a standard of care for HIV-associated wasting throughout the entire country (not only in the major metropolitan areas). Over fifty studies on anabolic steroids for HIV therapy have been conducted. Institutions like the AIDS Clinical Trials Group (ACTG), National Institutes of Health, University of California at Los Angeles, San Francisco, and Berkeley and several medical groups around the country have taken the lead in this search for validating data.

- Women and children suffer the most from misunderstandings about the use of anabolic steroids for effective wasting therapy. Some anabolic agents like the oral anabolic steroid oxandrolone (Oxandrin), which has very low androgenic potential, can be safely and effectively administered to women and children. However,

it is very expensive, so many HIV(+) people must turn to compassionate-use programs. The compassionate-use program for Oxandrin (made by BioTechnology General) is good. The injectable anabolic steroid nandrolone decanoate has been shown to be safe and effective in doses lower than men receive in a study with women who have 5 percent or more weight loss. We have also heard that some HIV(+) women are using oxymetholone (Anadrol) at 25 mg. per day with success.

- PoWeR strongly advocates legislating easier access to anabolic steroids as medicines. The Anabolic Steroid Control Act of 1990, while well intentioned, took these valuable and relatively nontoxic medicines, and categorized them as Code III, which means that distribution is strictly monitored by the Drug Enforcement Administration (DEA). In some states this means a doctor has to write a triplicate prescription that goes into DEA records. This makes doctors apprehensive about prescribing anabolic steroids, even for serious medical conditions. The Code III status and the publicity that grew around the law created an image that anabolic steroids are off-limits for any but rare medical uses, and that they are much more dangerous and toxic than they actually are when used in the correct medical context. Some physicians still think that they may lose their licenses if they prescribe anabolic steroids to their HIV(+) patients. While it is not legal to prescribe them for cosmetic or athletic uses, anabolic steroids can be prescribed in an off-label manner for muscle wasting diseases like AIDS and multiple sclerosis, and autoimmune diseases like lupus and rheumatoid arthritis. Anabolic steroids should also be considered for their therapeutic value for many other diseases, especially diseases that involve the immune system. As is true with many other diseases, anabolic steroids that are beneficial for AIDS wasting therapy are much less toxic than the majority of AIDS medications.

- Some doctors have actually said that providing appropriate anabolic steroid therapies such as testosterone replacement for hypogonadal patients, which may increase the patient's sex drive, is unethical due to the risk of spreading the HIV virus. HIV(+) individuals may die from wasting because of this kind of attitude. Safe sex has nothing to do with sex drive, but a lot to do with education. Sex drive is an integral part of the quality of life and the expression of love that all people need to lead fulfilled lives. Homophobia and sex-phobia have no place in medical practice.

- Studies are showing that specific anabolic steroids, unlike anti-inflammatory corticoid steroids, which exhibit specific immuno-suppressive effects, may improve important components of immune competence, like the CD8 T cells,[1] which appear to increase the potential for survival in AIDS.[2] Previous non-HIV(+) studies have shown that nandrolone can improve natural killer-cell activity.[3] Perhaps this is one reason why we have seen a significant reduction in opportunistic infections when HIV(+) people are given appropriate anabolic steroid therapy.

- Anabolic steroids also have other immune-modulating properties that might benefit autoimmune diseases like rheumatoid arthritis, lupus, and colitis. Studies with male and female HIV(+) individuals have begun to detail the effects anabolic steroids have on immune function in HIV. Some of them look not only at lean body mass,

but what effects other variables like proper nutrition and supervised weight training will have, too.

- Anabolic steroids, even though they are relatively economical and effective, have only recently begun to be included in any city, county, or state drug assistance programs available to the indigent or those with limited income. Costs for the two most commonly prescribed injectable steroids are very low. Testosterone cypionate can cost as little as $32 dollars per month, and nandrolone decanoate $125 per month for appropriate doses. However, only people who can afford them or who have insurance and a progressive doctor are accessing this treatment. Some HIV(+) people are forced to buy potentially dangerous counterfeit anabolic steroids from underground dealers (with no medical supervision) because of their doctor's lack of support when they ask for testosterone or other anabolic steroids. However, Megace, a very problematic drug that is not effective for increasing healthy weight, is still included in many drug assistance programs.

- Anabolic steroids are available at a low cost and over the counter in most third-world countries. This treatment option is one of the few which does not have to be imported from the industrialized world, and third-world countries are suffering the greatest increase in HIV infections, and without being able to afford the newest drugs. However, in my travels abroad, I have seen that Megace is still the number one drug used for wasting and that many physicians in other countries are afraid of anabolic steroid therapy.

5

Megace – The Wrong Drug
by James Brockman

One of the most commonly used drugs for treatment of AIDS-related weight loss is megestrol acetate, which is sold as the brand name Megace by Bristol-Myers Squibb. Megace is a synthetic drug categorized as a gestagen, which is a class of drugs that mimic the actions of the naturally occurring female hormone progesterone. Originally the drug was developed to be an injectable contraceptive for women, but the drug has now found a role as a chemotherapeutic agent in the treatment of several cancers in women and men, such as cancers of the breast, uterus, and prostate. Two commonly observed side effects of Megace, increased appetite and weight gain,[5] prompted its current use for AIDS-wasting.

The effects of progesterone and other gestagens, like Megace, on appetite and energy metabolism, are well known. Gestagens induce increased food intake by direct stimulation of the appetite centers in the brain.[6] They also improve the efficiency of food energy used to produce new tissue; this effect of gestagens on increasing weight is seen even when gestagen-induced increase in food intake is prevented by restricting calories to maintenance levels.[10] So much for the good points.

What Kind of Weight Gain?

The problem with the weight gained from Megace is that it is primarily fat and water weight, with little lean tissue increase.[7][8] Through interactions with mineral corticoid receptors in the kidneys, specific metabolites of Megace promote retention of water.[9] In addition, some studies have shown that Megace increases the number of fat cells as well as their size.[10] This is exactly what someone who is wasting or has lipodystrophy doesn't want. We should be clear that the focus of just putting weight on HIV(+) individuals is inappropriate. Studies are conclusive that survival is correlated with lean body mass, not total weight or fat weight. So if you want to be fat and hungry, take Megace, but do not expect to gain much muscle or live any longer.

Many Side Effects

Megace has almost too many side effects to list. For both men and women the most commonly observed side effect is loss of libido.[11] When Megace was used as a female contraceptive, it worked too well. All the women lost their fertility, but they lost their normal sex drive too! Megace interacts with the progesterone receptors in the hypothalamus to inhibit gonadotropin release in both sexes. Gonadotropins stimulate testosterone production, and testosterone is necessary for a healthy sex drive in both men and women. The end result of lower gonadotropins in men is not only lower testosterone production, and lower libido, but also testicular atrophy. In other words, the testicles shrivel up. Finally, low plasma testosterone levels are bad for HIV(+) men and women because they are associated with a weakened immune system and the loss of muscle tissue.

Because Megace and/or its metabolites have glucocorticoid activity,[9] Megace is also potentially immunosuppressive. Glucocorticoids are well known to inhibit proliferation of white blood cells including T cells, and weaken the body's response to infection, as well as slow the healing process. Furthermore, a glucocorticoid responsive element has been identified in the RNA of the HIV virus, so it is possible that Megace could have a direct effect on stimulating viral replication.[12] Other side effects related to the cortisol-like activity of Megace are glucose intolerance, full-blown diabetes,[13] and suppression of the hypothalamic-pituitary-adrenal (HPA) axis.[9] Resistance to cortisol is common in HIV, and withdrawal from Megace therapy could result in a dangerous state of adrenal deficiency. These conditions are associated with the later stages of HIV in cytokine-related wasting, so it makes little sense to use a drug that has the potential to make the complications of HIV infection even worse. Other problems seen with Megace include thrombosis (blood clots),[14] carpal tunnel syndrome,[15] and peripheral neuropathy.

Conclusions

When it comes to gaining muscle to rebuild a body weakened by AIDS, Megace cannot begin to stack up to anabolic steroids. While some people assert that Megace has a role as an appetite stimulant, there are other substances, like Marinol, that work with far fewer side effects. If your doctors are not yet aware of the benefits of Marinol and anabolic steroids, and the problems associated with Megace, work to educate them, and be sure to ask questions if they tell you they would like to prescribe Megace for you. After all, your choice of therapies is up to you.

6

Bioelectrical Impedance Analysis (BIA) and AIDS

by Nelson Vergel

Total Body Weight Does Not Tell Us Enough

Many medical doctors do not know about the use of a powerful, simple, and inexpensive tool to help assess their HIV(+) patients' health. As an HIV(+) patient, I have always been amazed that some doctors are only concerned about total body weight to assess whether a person is wasting or not. It is well known that although total body weight may not change for years after HIV infection, body composition changes even at asymptomatic stages. Lean body mass tends to decrease while fat and water weight tend to compensate for that decrease. Once lean body mass decreases to values close to 54 percent of normal, death occurs regardless of the cause.[16] A person could show signs of wasting even if his or her body weight is unchanged. I remember how some of my friends who are now dead used to argue that their weight had not changed at all, even though I could easily see their deterioration.

A simple technique called bioelectrical impedance analysis (BIA) can answer questions which cannot be answered with the common practice of putting a patient on a scale as soon as his or her name is called in a doctor's office.

One study showed that BIA indeed may be more useful for early detection of occult wasting in persons with HIV/AIDS in comparison to the normally used weight-for-height methods.[17]

BIA – Easy to Use and Covered by Insurance

BIA takes only a few minutes to determine a patient's body composition. It is accepted as a means for measuring nutritional status and body cell mass, and has been validated for this purpose in AIDS patients.[20] [18] [19] It is also reimbursable to doctors by insurance companies. Four self-adhering electrodes are attached to the subject's wrist and ankle on the same side of the body. A painless alternating current of 800 micro-amps at 50 kilohertz is then introduced. Electric current conductance is greater in lean tissue, as it contains most of the water-conducting electrolytes and cell mass in the body. Fat tissue, because of its lower water content, is less conductive.

Once the impedance measurements of resistance and reactance are made, a third number, the phase angle alpha can be calculated. From these three numbers, plus the patient's height, weight, sex, and age, it is also possible to estimate body cell mass, fat-free mass, and other body parameters. Body cell mass is the metabolically active tissue in the body, including muscle and organ tissues, and intracellular water. Lean body mass (LBM) includes body cell mass, along with extracellular water and bone. Note that lean body mass consists of more than just muscle tissue, and that many times patients and clinicians make a mistake assuming that lean body mass means muscle. Realize that BIA is less accurate in measurement of fat mass. For instance, if one is dehydrated from drinking coffee or as a result of a good workout, the measurement of fat can be highly inaccurate.

Phase Angle Alpha May Predict Survival Better Than T Cells

An interesting German study of seventy-five patients found that phase angle alpha predicted three-year survival better than CD4 T-cell count or any of several other measurements tested.[20] Body cell mass, serum cholesterol, CD4 count, and serum albumin were predictive to a lesser degree, while age, weight, serum protein, and serum triglycerides were not statistically significant in predicting survival.

The study analysis showed that patients with median phase angle alpha of 5.46 degrees had a somewhat greater than 50 percent survival over 1000 days. (The mean -1 standard deviation phase angle for 340 healthy control subjects was 5.6 degrees). Those at the 25th percentile – phase angle 4.87 degrees – which means that 25 percent of the patients in the study had a lower phase angle and 75 percent had a higher phase angle, had about 15 percent survival. For those at the 75th percentile (phase angle 5.96 degrees), survival was better than 80 percent. Until there is more definitive information, it may be reasonable to accept improvement in the phase angle obtained from BIA as an indicator of improved health. (I note that phase angle alpha's importance is still not proven.)

While there are several machines that employ impedance technology to measure body composition, the BIA machines that are used most often in clinical practice are manufactured by RJL Systems (33955 Harper Ave, Clinton Township, MI 48035, 800-528-4513). You can also visit their website for a great description of the technology: http://www.rjl-systems.com/research/fundamentals.html. They make a hand-held analyzer, a desktop model and a fully computerized version. A comprehensive weight, diet and exercise software program is included with each system. All of their BIA machines and corresponding software cost under $6,000. Many non-profit agencies, like the Montrose Clinic in Houston, provide free BIA to HIV(+) clients. Check your local HIV/AIDS organizations for more information. For more information about where to have BIA testing in the United States, visit http://www.medibolics.com/BIAcontacts.htm.

If you have your height, weight, desired weight (normal for your height and a BMI of 21 to 25 kg./m sq.) you can input this data along with the reductance and reactance to get your body composition in graphic format by visiting: http://interactive.rjlsystems.com

This article was reprinted with permission from: *Medibolics*, Volume 1, number 4.

7

Appetite Stimulation: Megace, Medicinal Marijuana, and Marinol
by Nelson Vergel and Michael Mooney

Food intake is critically important for building and maintaining lean body mass. Many people with HIV still experience loss of appetite or nausea that prevents them from having adequate food intake. That's why appetite stimulants can be an important part of the optimal approach to increasing lean body mass in HIV. However, all appetite stimulants are not equal in their effects on your overall health and well-being. The first drug used for appetite in the early years of AIDS was Megace. The previous chapter showed us that Megace should probably be relegated to the status of the problematic dinosaur drug that it is.

AIDS researcher Dr. Marc Hellerstein conducted a study to see if he could mitigate the negative effects that Megace has on body composition by providing testosterone to males at 200 mg. every two weeks with a standard 800 mg. daily dose of Megace. What he found was that even testosterone's powerful effect on metabolism could not inhibit the negative effects that Megace has, such as increasing body fat and decreasing libido.

Marijuana

We support the political battle to legalize marijuana for medical purposes. It provides significant unique benefits for people with cancer, HIV, glaucoma, and other serious medical problems. Our main concern about marijuana use is the damage that marijuana smoke can cause to lungs, just as any kind of smoke can damage lung tissues. While marijuana is known to be quite effective for improving appetite and reducing nausea, marijuana smoke contains over four hundred unusual compounds, including fungi and carcinogens. HIV(+) people who smoke marijuana have been documented to have an increased incidence of both fungal infections in the lungs and bacterial pneumonia.[21]

Furthermore, studies have shown that HIV(+) people who smoke marijuana may progress towards AIDS more rapidly, with a tendency towards increased opportunistic infections, including Kaposi's Sarcoma.[21 22 23] Smoking marijuana has also been shown to significantly reduce the ability of the immune components in the lungs to kill fungi, bacteria, and tumor cells, as well as decrease the lung tissue's ability to produce protective cytokines.[24]

While marijuana can also contain herbicides that are immunosuppressive, perhaps most problematic is the fact that marijuana contains about 30 percent more tar than tobacco, and marijuana smoking can decrease blood oxygen by about 50 percent more than tobacco.[25] Cancer thrives in low oxygen environments, so the tar and cancer-promoting potential of tobacco smoke should make any HIV(+) person avoid smoking marijuana. Therefore, if you do choose to use marijuana to increase appetite or reduce nausea, eat it, do not smoke it.

Marinol

Marinol (dronabinol) (www.marinol.com) is the other well-known oral pharmaceutical appetite stimulant that is prescribed for HIV. Chemically, it is a pure version of the most well known active ingredient in marijuana, called THC (delta-9-tetrahydra-cannabinol). Marinol can be prescribed by the doctor in three different dosages (2.5, 5, and 10 mg. capsules), so you can titrate the dosage to maximize benefits while minimizing the rather benign side effects that can occur, including sleepiness, thinking abnormalities, and euphoria (not a bad side effect).

In studies, Marinol treatment significantly improved appetite in people with HIV, while trends toward improved body weight and mood, and decreases in nausea and vomiting were also seen.[26] (Marinol has been approved to treat nausea in cancer.) It can however, take from twenty to forty minutes to get enough absorption of the drug in the bloodstream to feel the benefits. That is why it is generally agreed that if you are having severe nausea that is unpredictable, you may want to use one of the standard anti-emetics (i.e., Zofran), because they can work more quickly. However, if your nausea is predictable (as when Crixivan is taken on an empty stomach), you should consider Marinol.

Marinol has not been observed to decrease sex drive, decrease testosterone, or cause any of the adverse effects produced by Megace. However, there are a few things you should know when starting this therapy so that benefits can be maximized while minimizing side effects.

If you are considering starting Marinol to improve your appetite, it is generally recommended that you begin on a Friday night so that you have the weekend to acclimate to the effects of the drug, in case you do experience side effects. For most people, side effects subside within three days.

Most physicians will start you at 2.5 mg. twice a day, to be taken 1 hour before lunch and 1 hour before dinner. If side effects, like feeling "stoned," do not decrease during the first three days, the dosage should be reduced to 2.5 mg. once per day, usually taken 1 hour before dinner. This can also make it easier to sleep after dinner.

We have also known a few rare people for whom the 2.5 mg. dose is too much. They poke a hole in the capsule with a pin and squeeze out half of the dose. This usually gives them the right dose for improved appetite and more restful sleep.

The appetite-stimulating effect can last for over ten hours, so you will probably have a good dinner and wake up feeling hungry for breakfast, too. We also tell PoWeR clients who want to start this therapy to try not to eat junk food when their appetite increases. Make sure to stock your kitchen cupboards with nutritious high-protein snacks so that you have healthy bodybuilding foods handy when this happens. Marinol will help you gain good-quality lean body mass optimally if it is combined with a healthy, whole-foods diet that is high in protein, regular exercise as weight training, and hormonal therapies like testosterone, when appropriate. With the greater appetite that Marinol can give you, if you do not lift weights to stimulate muscle growth and burn calories you may very well increase your body fat instead of muscle.

Marinol Reclassified

In many states, in the summer of 1999, Marinol was re-classified from a Code II drug, which can require triplicate prescriptions, to Code III, which requires no triplicate, and can be called in to the pharmacy.

Easy Access

While we wait for legalization of medical marijuana, Marinol is easily accessed because it can be paid for by insurance, Medicaid, most state drug assistance programs, and by Roxane Laboratories' Compassionate Use Program, 800-274-8651.

8

How Do Anabolic Steroids Work?
by Michael Mooney and Nelson Vergel

Anabolic-androgenic steroids are synthetic analogs of the natural androgenic male hormone called "testosterone," which is produced primarily in the testes in males and in the ovaries in females. There are other kinds of steroids that have very different effects in the body – such as adrenal androgens, like the popular dietary supplement DHEA, and glucocorticoid steroids like cortisol. Many of the anabolic-androgenic steroids were synthesized in the 1950s in an effort to deliver a more optimum protein tissue-building (anabolic) effect with less of the potential masculinizing (androgenic) or feminizing (estrogenic) effects produced by the normal metabolism of testosterone. Testosterone metabolizes in the body into numerous compounds. However, two of its metabolites are important to discuss as they are related to reducing some of the possible side effects that testosterone can cause.

Testosterone converts into small amounts of "dihydro" testosterone (DHT), which promotes androgenic (masculine) effects in the body, and estrogen, which promotes feminizing effects. Both these effects are needed for normal optimum health, however an overabundance of them can cause significant side effects.

Too much of the androgenic effect in the body can increase problems like hair loss, and can stimulate the growth of tissues that are dense with cells that are sensitive to androgens, such as prostate

tissue. This may result in enlargement of the prostate. The molecular configuration of several of the anabolic steroids purposefully reduces their androgenic effects when the steroid is metabolized to its dihydro form. Some of the anabolic steroids are actually derived from dihydrotestosterone, but their molecular configuration is altered to reduce androgenic effects.

Unique molecular configurations of some steroids also thwart their conversion to estrogen, which reduces potential feminizing effects. Feminizing effects include the growth of breast tissue, a condition called "gynecomastia." The desired anabolic effects of the steroids are elicited by the action of the steroids on androgen receptors in muscle tissue. The steroid binds to the receptor and is carried to the nucleus of the cell where it tells the DNA in the cell to transcribe the steroid's message onto messenger-RNA (mRNA). The mRNA then delivers its message to the muscle cells and this causes a response in the cells that results in increased protein synthesis, which causes hypertrophy (growth) of the cells and the muscle tissue that the cells make up.

The different molecular configurations of the various anabolic steroids cause significantly different cellular responses, and even a subtle change of one atom can elicit a unique response for a specific steroid. That is why each steroid has distinct characteristics that make it more appropriate for specific therapeutic uses.

It should also be noted that anabolic steroids, in general, are hematopoietic (blood building) agents; they increase hemoglobin (red blood cell) production and hematocrit (blood cell volume).

INJECTABLE STEROIDS

Testosterone

Testosterone is the primary androgenic/anabolic ster_____ bodies of men and _____en.
Nor_____ are
abc_____The
M_____total
t_____ieral-
l_____is per
_____it usu-
_____normal
_____testos-
_____logically
_____y ranges
_____nen. For
_____and 1.28
_____" because
_____so it is free
_____als the cells
_____o note that
_____eclines with
_____ral diseases,
including HIV.

The two equivalent forms of injectable testosterone we recommend are the oil-based products, testosterone enanthate or testosterone cypionate. Testosterone enanthate is sold in the U.S. as a trade-name product, Delatestryl. Testosterone cypionate is sold as a trade-name product, Depo-Testosterone. These products come in various 1 mL, 5 mL, and 10 mL vials that contain 200 mg. per mL (milliliter).

The most economical version is the generic 10 mL multiple dose vial. Prices have varied considerably in recent years, but they are not high compared to many other medications, such as the antiviral drugs used for HIV.

Frequency of Administration – Testosterone (Once per Week)

While directions for the administration of both forms of testosterone often indicate to doctors that administration should be as infrequent as every two or three weeks, studies of the pharmacokinetics of these drugs show that this is inappropriate information if the most consistent blood levels of the drugs are desired. We should note that we constantly hear people complain of a large decrease in energy, libido, clarity of thought and mood by the time the two-or-more-week administration occurs.

One study stated that 140 mg. of testosterone cypionate and testosterone enanthate produced similar blood levels after injection, and stated that heightened blood levels decreased to basal levels by day ten. This means that the amount of testosterone in the blood was equal to what was there before the drug was administered.[27] With higher doses the duration appears to increase a little, as another study indicated that with an injection of 200 mg. of testosterone cypionate blood levels declined to basal levels by days thirteen to fourteen.[28]

Looking at the following chart, it is easy to see why a person would feel a large decline in energy, libido, stamina, mood, and overall quality of life with two-or-more-week dosing, so we urge the physician to consider adjusting dosing strategies. We believe that the patient will experience the greatest quality of life improvements when the cypionate and enanthate esters of testosterone are administered once every seven days.

We also suggest that forms of testosterone not currently available in the United States – like Sustanon, which is a long-acting testosterone blend,

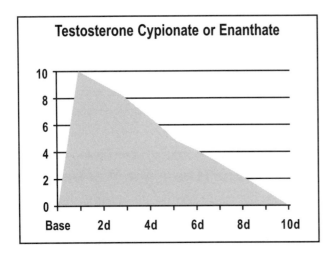

Testosterone Cypionate or Enanthate

Source: Schulte-Beerbuhl, 1980[27]
Blood Level versus Time in Days

with what appears to be a more consistent release (less peak and trough effect) than cypionate/enanthate – be investigated.

Testosterone is also available in the United States as an oil-based propionate, and a water-based suspension. Both of these forms are short acting and not desirable for our purposes.

Nandrolone Decanoate (Deca Durabolin)

Nandrolene decanoate is a "best" anabolic steroid for men because it has less potential for androgenic or estrogenic side effects than testosterone,[29] yet one comparison study showed that it has more anabolic potential than testosterone at lower doses. (See the comparison below.) Nandrolone, like other anabolic steroids, is not, however, suitable as a substitute for testosterone for the treatment of testosterone deficiency, as it does not produce the effects on libido, quality of life and physical hardiness that testosterone itself does. In truth, only testosterone itself is appropriate for testosterone replacement therapy.

Nandrolone's decreased androgenic potential means that there is less chance that it will promote hair loss or enlargement of the prostate than testosterone. This is partly because testosterone's 5-alpha reduced metabolite, called dihydrotestosterone, is more androgenic than nandrolone's 5-alpha reduced metabolite, called dihydronandrolone.[29] Because of its lower androgenic potential, nandrolone may also be used at low doses by women who are experiencing severe weight loss.

Nandrolone is a nor-testosterone, which means that there is no carbon at the 19 position of the molecule. This prevents the binding of the enzyme aromatase, which converts testosterone into estrogen. While some textbooks say that this means that nandrolone should not convert to estrogen at all, nandrolone has been shown to convert to estrogen at a rate of approximately 20 percent as much as testosterone does at therapeutic doses.[30] Therefore, nandrolone has significantly less potential to cause estrogen-related side effects such as gynecomastia (breast growth) than testosterone in men. Reduced potential for androgenic and estrogenic effects, along with its high anabolic potential makes nandrolone a very good steroid to combine with testosterone for higher-dose anabolic therapy.

Nandrolone probably converts to estrogen, not through the action of aromatase, but through the action of organic acids or alkalines in the body that act on nandrolone after it is converted to its 1-beta hydroxylated derivative. This means that estrogen inhibitors like Arimidex, which decrease the activity of aromatase, may not stop nandrolone from aromatizing to estrogen.

Frequency of Administration – Nandrolone (Once per Week)

Pharmacokinetic studies with nandrolone decanoate also show that it is better to administer it on a weekly basis rather than biweekly or monthly, if the most consistent blood levels of the steroid are desired. While blood levels of nandrolone decanoate begin to rise in several hours, its six-day half-life is about 20 percent longer than the half-life for testosterone enanthate or cypionate.[31] Note: The dosing information on the package insert for nandrolone decanoate recommends weekly administration. The dosing instructions in the package inserts for testosterone cypionate and enanthate are inadequate.

Oil-based injectable anabolic steroids are somewhat preferable to any oral steroid because they are not liver toxic.[32][33] The main reason that orals may be preferred is because some people have a strong aversion to injections and some doctors are reluctant to prescribe injectable drugs for self-administration.

Generic nandrolone decanoate and the trade-name product Deca Durabolin are sold as single dose vials in three different concentrations – 50 mg., 100 mg., or 200 mg. per mL. The most economical product contains 200 mg. per mL.

The Pool Effect

After several injections, long-acting injectable oil-based steroids like testosterone enanthate, testosterone cypionate, and nandrolone decanoate can accumulate in the muscle tissue around the injection site in a pool. This pooling can create a longer duration of release of the steroid, which may lengthen the net lifespan of the drug in the body to some extent. Even when this is taken into account, we suggest that once-a-week administration is best to maintain the most consistent blood level of the drug.

Comparing Anabolic Effect – Nandrolone versus Testosterone

While there have been no controlled comparative studies of nandrolone decanoate and testosterone in HIV(+) people, studies so far suggest that at a dose of 100 mg. per week, nandrolone produces more lean tissue growth than testosterone. For instance, in Dr. Julian Gold's study of wasting men, 100 mg. of nandrolone every two weeks caused a lean tissue gain of 6.6 pounds in sixteen weeks,[34] while Coodley's study on wasting men showed that 200 mg. of testosterone every two weeks produced no net gain after twelve weeks.[35] Gold's study did include weight training, though, and weight training

appears to roughly double the anabolic effect of anabolic steroids according to Dr. Bhasin's high-dose testosterone study.[36]

Perhaps more compelling is a comparative study of normal HIV(–) men that showed a significant weight gain with 100 mg. of nandrolone decanoate per week, but none with testosterone enanthate at 100 mg. In the same study, at 300 mg. of nandrolone and 300 mg. of testosterone, both steroids caused significant muscle gain, but there was a greater strength gain with testosterone.[37] (This suggests that testosterone induces specific natural neurochemical effects that influence physical strength that may be attenuated or devoid with nandrolone.)[38] There is nothing perfectly conclusive here, but this data does indicate that nandrolone probably does have more value as an anabolic agent than testosterone does at equal low-replacement-like doses. This supports our proposed use of nandrolone added to replacement testosterone to increase the net anabolic effect with less potential for the androgenic or estrogenic side effects that might happen with higher-than-replacement dose testosterone. However, testosterone appears to have its own unique functional effects on the nervous system.

Combining Testosterone with Nandrolone to Reduce Side Effects

We also suggest that physicians consider using a mixture of nandrolone decanoate and testosterone in equal lower doses to give some more sensitive hypogonadal men the full benefit of the androgenic properties of testosterone, but reduce the potential for its dose-related side effects. Testosterone's androgenic characteristics impart more energy, physical strength, libido, and anti-depressive effect than nandrolone, but there is more potential for hair loss, acne, irritability, and prostate growth with testosterone, especially with increasing doses.

Nandrolone appears to add relatively more anabolic activity with a reduced potential for side effects. We see physicians prescribe 50 to 100 mg. of testosterone with 50 to 100 mg. of nandrolone per week to men to obtain better overall lean tissue retention, energy, and quality of life than can be obtained by using testosterone or nandrolone alone. There is also less potential for hair loss and other side effects with this combination.

We sometimes hear men tell us how testosterone alone makes them feel less than optimal until nandrolone is added. We have seen low dose combinations of testosterone and nandrolone used by a significant number of men to produce optimal quality of life, and suggest that physicians consider this non-standard use.

ORAL STEROIDS AND RISK FACTORS

While oil-based injectable steroids like testosterone and nandrolone are not liver toxic,[32][33] oral steroids may be preferred by some people because they do not like injections. Liver toxicity is associated with oral steroids primarily because oral steroids are 17-alpha alkylated. If a non-alkylated steroid is taken orally it is broken down rapidly when it passes through the liver before it can create an effect in the muscle cells. This is the reason that common injectable steroids will not produce results if they are swallowed. Alkylating the steroid, however, slows the liver's inactivation of the molecule so that it is metabolized in secondary pathways that are less efficient. This can result in an alteration in liver cell function that may express itself as elevations in SGOT, SGPT, LDH, GGT and bilirubin blood tests that can indicate liver toxicity.

Oral steroids appear to increase the potential for cardiovascular risk because they lower HDL cholesterol and increase LDL cholesterol during use (but they are not generally known to increase total cholesterol). Lowered HDL and increased LDL are considered to be risk factors for cardiovascular disease. Whether their effect on HDL and LDL cholesterol actually increases cardiovascular risk is not clear, and there is little data in the medical literature that confirms that this effect does, of itself, cause adverse events. It is possible that any effect on HDL and LDL does not produce significant risk unless it is combined with other risk factors like high-fat, high-glycemic, hypercaloric diets, a lack of antioxidants in the diet, or genetic predisposition. However, the risk becomes more significant when we consider that a majority of the population is not disciplined in their dietary habits or nutrient intake.

On the other hand, oral steroids have the potential to decrease triglycerides by their action of increasing post-heparin triglyceride lipase activity in the liver.[34] In one recent study that looked at 57,000 people, elevated triglycerides were shown to be a significant risk factor for atherosclerosis, regardless of LDL.[40] This might suggest that oral steroids could reduce cardiovascular risk, but this generalization seems unlikely.

With oral steroids producing two seemingly contradictory effects on cardiovascular risk, much more needs to be studied before we can conclude what effect oral anabolic steroids have on the cardiovascular system. In the meantime, it is advisable to take precautions, such as maintaining a minimum optimal intake of vitamin E (400 IU, three times per day) and vitamin C (1,000 mg. three times per day) during any use of oral steroids to reduce the oxidation of LDL cholesterol that increases the potential for atherosclerosis. It also seems likely that the potential of both oral and injectable steroids to increase blood pressure could be their most important negative effect on cardiovascular risk.

Stanozolol (Winstrol)

Stanozolol is available for humans in the United States as a 2-mg. tablet. In both its injectable and oral forms it is 17-alpha alkylated, and therefore may present some burden to the liver, although studies on animals and humans suggest that any actual negative effect may be negligible at appropriate medical doses. Stanozolol has very low androgenic potential relative to its anabolic potential, and while some people seem to respond to it rather well, it is still considered in practical application by many people to be only a medium strength anabolic agent. At the same time, it is considered by some to be somewhat more effective than other relatively safe oral anabolic steroids, like oxandrolone and methenolone (trade-named Primobolan, sold in Europe and Mexico). Because stanozolol is a dihydrotestosterone-based molecule, it does not convert to estrogen, and does not increase water retention the way that steroids that convert to estrogen, like testosterone, can. Its potential for other side effects is also quite low. Its approved medical indication is for angioedema.

There has been one small study published on stanozolol used with HIV(+) males that showed good body weight gains with a relatively low dose of 6 to 12 mg. per day with no significant effect on the liver at this dose.[41] However, we have only heard reports of a few doctors prescribing stanozolol to HIV(+) men in the United States. We invite physicians to consider its use, as it is much less costly than oxandrolone. (See the comparison chart in Chapter 19, page XX.)

We have also seen 12 mg. of stanozolol per day appear to significantly reduce weight loss in HIV(+) men who were suffering from the catabolic effects of an infection or diarrhea. There is inference in the literature that this might be possible, as one comparison study showed that stanozolol was superior to several other steroids in inhibiting the catabolic effect of cortisone.[42 43]

Oxandrolone (Oxandrin)

Oxandrolone (www.oxandrin.com) is the only anabolic steroid that has been approved by the FDA for weight loss, so cautious doctors are more likely to prescribe it. It is a relatively safe oral steroid with a low potential for creating androgenic side effects. In fact, oxandrolone is so safe that it was prescribed for many years for male and female children with stunted growth (Turner's syndrome). It was removed voluntarily from the U.S. market in 1992 when the political climate and the laws regarding steroids changed, but returned in 1995 to be sold to the HIV marketplace.

While some HIV studies show a good anabolic response to doses as low as 15 mg. per day, and anecdotal reports tell us that oxandrolone is an effective anabolic agent for some people at 20 mg. per day, doctors' anecdotes and one case review study tell us that some males have only a weak response at 20 mg. per day.[44] However, one controlled study showed that 20 mg. of oxandrolone per day combined with 100 mg. of testosterone enanthate per week and weight training produced considerable lean body mass gains.[45] We have seen oxandrolone produce much better results when it is combined with testosterone.

While promotional materials for Oxandrin state that it is "13 times as anabolic as testosterone," this is scientifically incorrect, and a misquote from the original literature. The original text that this phrase was taken from stated that oxandrolone is thirteen times as anabolic as it is androgenic,[46] and this number has only a very indirect relationship to testosterone's anabolic potential. Actually, these kinds of measurements, called disassociation ratios, are not considered to be scientifically credible by scientists like Dr. Charles Kochakian, the man known as the "father of anabolic steroids."[47] (This method employs the levator ani, a muscle that is not like other muscles in the body, in that it is dependent on androgens for normal function.) The truth is, while oxandrolone is the safest steroid for women and children that is available in the U.S., and can be quite effective for some males, it is probably the mildest of the anabolic steroids that are currently available. Because it is a dihydrotestosterone-based molecule it does not convert to estrogen or cause estrogen-related side effects.

While oxandrolone is promoted as being safe for the liver, all commonly available oral steroids have the potential to burden the liver. At the 1998 Geneva AIDS Conference, Dr. Carl Grunfeld noted that preliminary data on a recent large multi-site dose-ranging HIV study that looked at 20, 40 and 80 mg. of oxandrolone per day showed that at the 40 and 80 mg. doses oxandrolone produced elevated SGOT and SGPT, which can indicate liver toxicity. We have been surprised that a number of HIV(+) men have reported significant elevations of liver function tests with oxandrolone use. It is suspected that this happens because oxandrolone is metabolized in the same p450 3A4 liver enzyme pathway as protease inhibitors. This needs to be studied.

Although oxandrolone has been said to have no effect on testosterone production, it does attenuate the body's natural testosterone production, the same as all other effective anabolic steroids. At only 10 mg. per day, oxandrolone has been shown to reduce endogenous (the body's own) testosterone production by 62 percent.[33] All anabolic steroids that are effective have an effect on the body's natural testosterone production when given at "anabolic" doses.

Oxandrolone is currently priced at $535 per 100 tablets of 2.5 mg. and $1138 per 100 tablets of 10 mg. in the U.S., which makes cost a consideration. (The retail price before 1992, when oxandrolone, then known as "Anavar," was removed from the U.S. market, was about 20 cents per tablet.) However, BTG, oxandrolone's manufacturer in the U.S., has a very helpful patient assistance program.

Oxymetholone (Anadrol-50)

Oxymetholone is thought to be the most powerful oral anabolic steroid, and although it has a reputation among bodybuilders as being one of the most liver toxic, this is controversial. Oxymetholone is typically prescribed in HIV in doses of 50 mg. (one tablet), 100 mg., and 150 mg. per day, and the fact that the tablet doses are so high may account for some of its reputation for toxicity. While oxandrolone and stanozolol are reputed to have much less potential for toxicity, they have historically been studied at 5- to 20-mg. doses, so credible comparisons with oxymetholone are difficult, as toxicity is a dose-related effect. It is likely that if oxandrolone and stanozolol were compared with oxymetholone at similar higher doses for the typically long periods of time that oxymetholone has been studied, their potential for toxicity would be more apparent. Indeed, as was noted earlier, there was evidence of liver toxicity in the first HIV study of oxandrolone at 40 and 80 mg., but not at 20 mg.

At oxymetholone's currently recommended daily dose of 100 mg., which is considerably higher than is necessary to promote muscle growth, oxymetholone can cause water retention, high blood pressure, hair loss, acne, increase in blood clotting time, mood changes, increases in liver function tests and most of the other side effects that are possible with high doses of other anabolic steroids. We also know HIV(+) men who have used oxymetholone at 100 and 150 mg. per day who have experienced no significant side effects, but tremendous muscle growth, improved hematocrit, and increased energy and libido. An effective dose of oxymetholone can be much lower than the 100 mg. standard prescription dose, and at an individually determined lower dose many HIV(+) people report strong effects on muscle growth without problems. Recently, we have been surprised to find that some HIV(+) women are using oxymetholone at as much as 25 mg. per day for good effects on lean weight gain, seemingly without significant masculinizing effects.

While oxymetholone does not convert to estrogen because of its saturated a-ring, gynecomastia (feminized breasts) has been seen in males using oxymetholone, but this generally only occurs if it is combined with growth hormone or testosterone, either of which can cause gynecomastia by themselves. Used alone, we have seen oxymetholone cause gynecomastia to shrink quickly, probably because oxymetholone can exert inhibitory, anti-estrogenic effects on hormone-responsive breast tissue.

One caveat about oxymetholone is the potential to cause a decrease in glutathione production in the liver. One in vitro (test tube) study showed that while testosterone, nandrolone, and stanozolol did not cause a significant decrease in liver cell glutathione, oxymetholone did.[32] How significant this effect may be in humans is not clear; but it does provide a rationale for those who take oxymetholone or any oral steroid to take the dietary supplements that increase glutathione production and protect the liver, including glutamine, N-acetyl cysteine, selenium, alpha lipoic acid, silymarin, and Vitamin C. (Read more about these supplements in Chapter 20, *Orthomolecular Nutrition*.)

GELS, CREAMS AND PATCHES

Other forms of testosterone include transdermal products. "Transdermal" means that the steroid is delivered by being absorbed through the skin (dermis). It is dissolved in a carrier and ideally placed in contact with areas of the body where there is thin skin and a rich blood supply, so that absorption is optimum. Regardless, this is not a very efficient way to deliver testosterone, as dermal absorption can be quite poor. Testosterone patches were first sold as a patch that was applied directly to the scrotum. This product was called Testoderm, and contained either

4 or 6 mg. of testosterone per patch per twenty-four hours. Androderm and Testoderm TTS are other patches that are made to allow application to other body parts. Androderm comes in 2.5-mg. or 5-mg. strengths. Testoderm TTS contains 5 mg. per patch. We do not generally recommend patches to men because they do not deliver enough testosterone to promote increases in muscle mass that are comparable to the effects of injectable testosterone for men. They can, however, supply enough testosterone to provide some men with an improved sense of well being, more energy and an increased sex drive. Women require much less testosterone to experience benefits, so patch products may be more beneficial to women.

Gels are generally more effective than patches because they can be made to deliver more testosterone. Creams, that are basically similar to gels in effect, are also available. Androgel, made by UNIMED Pharmaceuticals, comes in ready-made pouches containing 25-mg. or 50-mg. doses. Testim, the next generation gel made by Auxilium Pharmaceuticals, comes in unit dose resealable tubes containing 50 mg. Gels and creams made at compounding pharmacies, such as Applied Pharmacy Services (formerly GulfSouth) at (www.appliedpharamacyrx.com), Kronos Pharmacy, Women's International Pharmacy (http://www.womensinternational.com/about.html) and others can be compounded to contain much higher doses. Most men seem to prefer gels, while women seem to prefer creams. We do not recommend gels, patches or creams to men who are losing weight and need the power that injectable testosterone can deliver. Again, these products may deliver enough testosterone for women to experience significant benefits.

9

First Placebo-Controlled Steroid Study Suggests Improved Immune Function

by Michael Mooney

When Nelson and I started our work together in June 1994, after the late Dr. Dullnig passed away, we were a decided minority in the world of AIDS that was, for the most part, unreasonably prejudiced against the medical use of anabolic steroids. Back then there were only two small publications on steroid use for HIV. One was a small study conducted by Dr. Julian Gold in Australia using nandrolone decanoate, and the other a patient chart review published by Dr. Walter Jekot. Many people thought we were crazy radicals who were just "steroid pushers." Then, in 1996, came Dr. Bucher's groundbreaking placebo-controlled study that showed that anabolic steroids could not only help HIV(+) people gain weight safely, but might even benefit the immune system.

At the Vancouver XI International Conference on AIDS, on July 9, 1996, Dr. Gary Bucher of Chicago's Center for Special Immunology presented the first placebo-controlled study of the anabolic steroid nandrolone decanoate (Deca Durabolin) with seventy-three HIV(+) people over twelve weeks. Results showed why steroids can be valuable for wasting therapy and supported the assertion that anabolic steroids are not immunosuppressive, but may potentiate important barometers of immune competence. There was a significant increase in lean body mass, and there was a significant increase in the number of CD8 T cells averaging 153 points. These facts are important because optimal lean body mass has a direct association with survival,[48] and while CD8s need much more investigation, some research does suggest that higher numbers of these cells may strongly correlate with survival.[49]

Although this study did not show what is considered to be a statistically significant change in CD4 count, there was no negative effect, and the trend line was moving up ever so slightly. There was no statistically significant change in viral load, but the trend line was moving down slightly. Hematocrit increased significantly.

Note that the dosage used in this study was rather low – 100 mg. of nandrolone decanoate per week.[50] For instance, a study directed by Dr. Fred Sattler, at the University of Southern California at Los Angeles, used 600 mg. of nandrolone per week.[3] This higher dose was studied because there is good reason to believe that it is much more effective for increasing lean body mass and that it is safe for this use. Because some of the progressive medical research community in the United States are aware of the safety and efficacy of correctly administered anabolic steroids, there are other studies in process that are using these higher doses.

Things to watch for in higher dose studies include noting whether the two slight trends of increasing CD4 cell counts and decreasing viral loads will increase, perhaps to the point of statistical significance. Additionally, the Sattler study employed controlled weight training, so considerably more lean body mass was gained with a higher steroid dose and the extra stimulation of weight training.

After the Vancouver AIDS Conference, protease inhibitor combos and other expensive medicines received international press, and justifiably so, but Dr. Bucher's groundbreaking anabolic steroid study received little coverage. It was not picked up by any newsletter from the major AIDS organizations that I am aware of, and I am convinced that this is due to politics. The misinformation about anabolic steroid safety and effectiveness has kept them in medical limbo in a community that continues to see our friends waste and die. The sad truth is that anabolic steroids, perhaps more than any other medication, can make wasting, and perhaps death from wasting, which has been a leading cause of death from AIDS in North America, a very rare occurrence. But steroids are still viewed as taboo by many doctors. Hopefully this attitude will change, as we learn the results of the numerous studies that will be completed in the future. We need to hear more of the safety and effectiveness of these inexpensive medicines.

10
Steroid Legality and the Physician
by Michael Mooney

The Anabolic Steroid Act of 1990 created grave misunderstandings, both for the public and for physicians trying to help their patients, about the legal status of steroids as medicines. This law states that androgenic-anabolic steroids cannot be prescribed for cosmetic or athletic purposes. But the impression it created was that steroids were off limits to everyone, and that they are basically illegal for any use. This is definitely not the case. To compound this climate of fear, it seems that when this law was passed in 1990, several of the more conservative regional governing medical organizations made an effort to make doctors uneasy, giving them the impression that they would become the object of scrutiny if they prescribed steroids at all. However, this attitude has fortunately been changing in recent years.

Testosterone and the androgenic-anabolic steroids have clear documentation that supports their medical use for numerous specific pathologies. These include various anemias, hypo-testosterone-mia (inadequate testosterone production), muscle wasting diseases, angioedema, phenylketonuria (inability to metabolize the amino acid phenylalanine), weight loss, leukemia, breast cancer, and some other cancers. The scientific literature also shows that anabolic steroids may be useful for treatment of autoimmune diseases, such as rheumatoid arthritis, multiple sclerosis, and lupus.

The physician who cares for HIV(+) patients has the legal right to prescribe anabolic steroids for medical use to any critically ill patient within the same specific guidelines that apply to numerous other medications used by critically ill patients. For instance, if a patient measures at the low end (or below) of normal total testosterone, or suffers from the symptoms of hypogonadism (low testosterone production), such as impotence, testosterone replacement is indicated. One study showed that the standard testosterone replacement dose of 100 mg. per week (or 200 mg. every two weeks) for HIV(–) men was inadequate for weight-gain in HIV(+) progressed men.[51] In HIV disease there is hormonal insensitivity, as was suggested by data provided in a study by Judith Rabkin, Ph.D., of New York, where she showed that HIV(+) hypogonadal men generally needed a higher testosterone replacement dose than the standard dose for HIV(–) hypogonadal men to experience the normal quality of life benefits. As described in Chapter 19, Dr. Rabkin found that her subjects needed to be given 400 mg. every two weeks to respond favorably.[52]

In 1988, frequently-published endocrinologist Dr. Adrian Dobs of Johns Hopkins noted that about 50 percent of HIV(+) men are hypogonadal.[53] Dr. Steven Grinspoon found a similar situation with women.[54] When we consider this and Dr. Rabkin's data, perhaps as much as half of HIV(+) men and women need replacement testosterone, and men may need doses of testosterone that will bring them into the high range of blood testosterone measurement or slightly above. The physician should measure testosterone, but also consider whether the patient is exhibiting the classic symptoms of hypotestosteronemia (fatigue, lack of libido, sexual dysfunction, depression, muscle loss, and lack of appetite) to determine whether it is appropriate to administer testosterone replacement therapy. Monitoring both the patient's subjective feelings about their symptoms and their testosterone blood levels two or three days after the fourth weekly injection will confirm whether the therapy is appropriate.

We also know knowledgeable doctors who do not measure testosterone because the measurements do not always mirror the patient's condition. Impotence, for instance, is a valid reason to prescribe testosterone, and we know doctors who prescribe testosterone for this indication when no weight loss is present. Often the person's response shows them that testosterone therapy is correct, regardless of the measurements.

Progressive Uses

The anabolic steroid analogs of testosterone, like nandrolone, oxandrolone, stanozolol, and oxymetholone are not appropriate for androgen replacement therapy by themselves, as they do not provide all of the characteristics that are necessary for normal androgen function. Their best use is as adjuncts to the use of testosterone as the fundamental androgen. They are generally used for improving lean body mass for people who have measurable loss of lean body mass; however, the most progressive physicians in several of the major metropolitan areas have been using anabolic steroids proactively for thin patients before wasting occurs to improve lean body mass so that there is a sufficient reserve of lean body mass in case the patient suffers an opportunistic infection and experiences a rapid loss of lean body

mass. This steroid-induced extra lean body mass can act as a buffer so that the patient doesn't ever fall into the danger zone as outlined by Dr. Donald Kotler, where he showed that loss of lean body mass to 54 percent of normal equals death.[55] An example of this would be a six-foot tall male who has always weighed 140 pounds. This person is below normal on the Metropolitan Life Insurance table. This person would have much better chances of surviving a catabolic (muscle-destroying) infection that might cause significant weight loss if he weighed 170 pounds. The primary consideration here is the person's overall health and ability to withstand infection-induced weight loss.

Cautious physicians are unlikely to employ the more controversial and aggressive uses of anabolic steroids if they think they may be challenged legally. These physicians may choose to restrict their use of anabolic steroids to oxandrolone combined with testosterone replacement, as oxandrolone is the only steroid that is specifically indicated for "failure to gain or maintain normal weight." However, in the major metropolitan areas, where numerous physicians are known to prescribe testosterone and anabolic steroids to hundreds or thousands of HIV(+) people, there is little likelihood of any legal problem, even though for steroids other than oxandrolone, weight gain is an off-label use. We know of doctors in every major city who employ anabolic steroids very progressively, sometimes using very high doses and unusual combinations of different steroids that they have learned to tailor for specific patient needs. We are unaware of any physician in the United States ever being reprimanded for prescribing anabolic steroids for legitimate use in HIV therapy.

The use of anabolic steroids is currently being investigated in over a dozen studies funded by government and medical agencies, so we are fast approaching the day when we will see the kind of broad range acceptance that will yield an understanding that testosterone and anabolic steroids are a major part of the standard of care for HIV and HIV-related wasting. We believe that any physician in this country can prescribe anabolic steroids within the context of the guidelines we feature in this book without repercussion from any government agency or medical board. After all, HIV is a critical illness.

11

An Initiative: New Directions for Wasting Research from Program for Wellness Restoration (PoWeR)

by Nelson Vergel and Michael Mooney

Program for Wellness Restoration (PoWeR) is the only community-based, national AIDS research organization that focuses on empowering HIV(+) people and their physicians with information about a comprehensive program to increase lean body mass for improved survival and immune function. Our unique program incorporates the use of enhanced nutrition, micronutrient supplementation, resistance weight training, and androgenic-anabolic steroids and other hormonal therapies.

We at PoWeR, the community of people with HIV and AIDS we serve, and the physicians and researchers we work with, have recognized for several years that the issues of quality of life and overall health addressed by our approach are crucial to people living with HIV and AIDS.

Program for Wellness Restoration has utilized over twelve years of real-world experience in designing anabolic steroid guidelines used to treat AIDS-associated wasting in clinical settings. Our guidelines are in use by over two hundred physicians and medical groups throughout this country and in Canada.

Several wasting-reversal or wasting-prevention studies are currently underway that use nandrolone decanoate, Megace and testosterone combinations, oxymetholone, oxandrolone, or Serostim. We think that it is time for the research community involved

in these studies to engage in an open dialogue to share experiences and maximize the use of resources without overlapping in their research efforts. We raise the challenge to the AIDS Clinical Trials Group, AMFAR, CRIA, and other organizations in the AIDS research community, to seize the initiative in this area and in a coordinated manner run community-based clinical trials to explore the intriguing possibilities raised by our twelve years of peer-driven experience.

Wasting is not a thing of the past, and research in this area should continue because even those people who benefit from the use of the new protease inhibitor combinations have a difficult time gaining back healthy lean body mass. Dr. Deeks of the University of California at San Francisco has shown that as much as 50 percent of the HIV population does not fully benefit from protease inhibitor therapy. As you will read, protease inhibitor combinations may increase weight, but the weight is primarily fat. There is also some data that suggests that at least 26 percent of the people are still losing lean body mass while on protease combination therapies.[56]

What has been done so far in the area of research about the clinical application of anabolic steroids for HIV disease? A few small studies show some promising results.

ANABOLIC HORMONES AND AIDS

As many of us know, we need a lot more controlled studies of anabolic steroid applications in AIDS than we have right now. However, as of early 1999 there have been several placebo-controlled anabolic steroid studies that compared one group of subjects who were using an anabolic steroid to another group of subjects who weren't. The trend continues as we are seeing other studies and publications of anecdotal experiences by more and more researchers and physicians around the world. A brief review of only a little of the data follows.

Testosterone Undecanoate

Jeantils (1993) published a small study in which oral testosterone undecanoate (available in Europe, but not in the U.S.) was given for two months to four HIV(+) patients at a dosage of 40 mg. three times daily.[57] No side effects were noted. Assessment of liver enzymes showed no disturbance. Weight increased by an average of 14.8 percent (11.2 lbs.). The average body mass index was increased by 13.5 percent. Blood albumin levels (a good marker for reduced wasting) increased by 18.4 percent. Beta-2 microglobulin (a marker for immune activation) decreased by 34 percent. Total lymphocytes increased by 9 percent (no subset given).

Winstrol (stanozolol)

A small study that used stanozolol, an oral anabolic steroid available in the U.S., was performed by Joseph Berger, M.D. (1993).[58] The study involved three HIV(+) males taking AZT with CD4 counts of 165 cells per cu mm, 39 cells per cubic millimeter, and 206 cells per cubic millimeter, respectively. Their creatine kinase (CK) values were abnormally low, which indicated signs of myopathy (muscle weakness). They had all lost over 10 percent of their normal body weight. They also showed signs of fatigue. Two were given stanozolol, 2 mg. orally three times per day for one month, and one required 4 mg. three times per day to effect a gain in weight. (Note: Illicit use doses for athletes can be much higher.) All three patients showed increased weight (e.g., 10.25 pounds average in ten weeks) and energy levels, with no significant side effects. No immunological markers were assessed, but quality of life (QOL) measures increased significantly.

Testosterone Enanthate

A study performed in 1993 by Judith Rabkin, Ph.D., and Richard Rabkin, M.D. at the New York State Psychiatric Institute was designed to determine whether testosterone therapy influences sexual dysfunction, mood, energy, and appetite among hypogonadal HIV(+) men with significant immune suppression (CD4 < 400 cells per mm).[59] Forty-one men entered the study and thirty-seven completed at least eight weeks of treatment. Hormones like LH, FSH, prolactin, and total serum testosterone were assessed at baseline along with immune parameters (T-cell panel, CBC, and others). Appetite, libido, mood, and energy improved significantly after the treatments (which consisted of biweekly injections of testosterone cypionate at a starting dose of 100 mg., increasing by 100 mg. up to 400 mg. at the end of the study). Only six subjects reported any side effects; among those were irritability (2), feeling hyper (2), feeling overly assertive (2), and hair loss (2). CD4 cell counts did not change significantly during the fifteen weeks of the study. No lean body mass measurements were taken. Dr. Judith Rabkin stated in personal correspondence that the HIV(+) hypogonadal men in her study appeared to need testosterone enanthate at a dose of 400 mg. every two weeks to get normal quality of life barometers. We revisit Dr. Rabkin's work in Chapter 19, *Anabolic Hormone Guidelines*, of this book, and discuss what appears to cause the need for higher testosterone replacement doses than what is standard for HIV(–) men.

Testosterone Combined with Nandrolone

Barry Chadsey, M.D., an HIV(+) Los Angeles physician, a former football player and bodybuilder, used anabolic steroids to treat the effects of wasting with over one hundred of his patients over nine years. Many of his patients gained twenty to thirty pounds.[60] He also saw significant improvements in certain T-cell counts in his patients. About three-quarters of his patients experienced increases in their CD8 counts and 40 percent experienced increases in CD4 counts. Dr. Chadsey was noted for using a cycling strategy with testosterone cypionate and nandrolone decanoate in a pyramid style escalating/de-escalating mode over twelve weeks, which is the format the PoWeR cycle is modeled after. (See the PoWeR cycle in Chapter 19.)

Similar benefits have also been reported in a paper published by Walter Jekot, M.D., a Los Angeles doctor who pioneered anabolic steroid therapy for AIDS.[61] Dr. Jekot emphasized that those patients who accompanied anabolic steroid treatment with the use of vitamin supplements, a nutrient-rich diet, and moderate resistance exercise seem to be the best responders.

Testosterone Enanthate

Notably, the first controlled study on high-dose testosterone enanthate supplementation with normal HIV(–) men was published in the *New England Journal of Medicine* on July 4, 1996.[62] This study employed 600 mg. of testosterone enanthate per week for ten weeks, and was controlled for weight training. Those who were given testosterone but did not lift weights at all gained more lean mass (7 lbs.) than those who trained with weights but were not given testosterone (4.4 lbs.). The testosterone group who didn't exercise also gained almost as much

strength as the group who only exercised. Those who lifted weights and were given testosterone gained almost twice as much lean mass as the testosterone with no exercise group, which amounted to over thirteen pounds, and experienced significantly greater increases in strength in the squat and bench press than the other groups. The authors detectecd no effect on behavior (no roid rage) or liver problems.

Comment: It is important to note that until the publication of this study the position of the conservative medical community was that testosterone alone or anabolic steroids in general haven't been proven to increase lean body mass or strength and shouldn't necessarily be used for HIV-associated wasting. This study makes obvious the fact that anabolic steroids do increase lean body mass, that supraphysiologic (very high) doses work better than lower doses like the 100 mg. per week that was used in many previous studies, and that including weight training produces significantly more increase in lean body mass.

Testosterone Combined with Nandrolone and Oxandrolone

A review study presented by Dr. Patricia Salvato of Houston's ONCOL Medical Group at the Second International Conference on Nutrition and HIV in Cannes, France, in April 1997, showed that twenty subjects who were using the PoWeR program, which consists of twelve weeks of high doses of nandrolone decanoate and testosterone cypionate (700 mg. per week total of the two compounds during the middle of the twelve weeks), effectively reversed wasting with an average weight gain of thirteen pounds (8.02 percent).[63] Serum albumin, a marker that decreases in wasting, increased by 23 percent. No liver toxicity or adverse effects were observed. Quality of life as assessed by a questionnaire was improved by 188.75 percent. Although other studies have shown benefit from the use of oxandrolone at 20 mg. per day, this study showed that 20 mg. per day of oxandrolone had very little effect (<1 percent weight increase) on reversing wasting in patients who had lost over 10 percent of their normal body weight. This study showed that adding 20 mg. per day of oxandrolone to the PoWeR cycle did not provide any additional benefit.

Oxandrolone

While studies on oxandrolone alone at 20 mg. per day have generally shown good gains in LBM, the tightly-controlled Strawford study showed that this dose of oxandrolone combined with testosterone at 100 mg. per week and weight training is perhaps an optimal way to employ oxandrolone. Subjects using this combination gained an average of 15.18 pounds of LBM.[64]

Nandrolone Decanoate

Dr. Julian Gold, et al., of Australia, reported in his sixteen-week study that even with very low dose nandrolone (100 mg. every two weeks), lean body mass and quality of life improved significantly (6.6 lbs.) in wasting-HIV patients with no negative effect on CD4 lymphocytes.[65] Dr. Gold was a trailblazer, as his study included nutritional assessment and suggestions for weight training before anyone else had done this. We applaud Dr. Gold.

As mentioned earlier, at the XI International AIDS Conference (Vancouver), Dr. Gary Bucher, of Chicago's Center for Special Immunology, presented his placebo-controlled study of the anabolic steroid nandrolone (Deca Durabolin) at 100 mg. per week for twelve weeks with seventy-three HIV patients.[66] This study showed excellent results, which supported the need for more studies with nandrolone decanoate.

At the Bethesda NIH Conference on May 20, 1997, Dr. Marc Hellerstein said that about 50 percent of his HIV patients in San Francisco do not produce adequate testosterone. His team concluded a study that employed nandrolone decanoate that showed an 11.88-pound increase in lean body mass in twelve weeks. Nandrolone decreased lipogenesis (fat generation) significantly (nutrients tended to contribute to lean tissue more than to fat tissue). Improvements in strength, endurance, and quality of life paralleled body composition changes.[67]

Dr. Fred Sattler of the University of Southern California at Los Angeles recently published the results of his high dose (600 mg. per week) nandrolone decanoate study that compared nandrolone alone to nandrolone with weight training with thirty HIV(+) males.[58] Both groups gained strength and muscle size, with the group that trained with weights gaining significantly more strength and LBM. This study showed that, even without weight training, high-dose nandrolone can increase LBM and muscle size and strength.

Testosterone Combined with Megace

Also at the Bethesda NIH Conference, Dr. Hellerstein presented the results of a study that investigated combining Megace (800 mg. per day) with testosterone (either a 200-mg. injection every other week or a Testoderm testosterone patch or placebo). He concluded that the great majority of weight gain in all the Megace-treated groups, with or without testosterone, was composed of fat.

Serostim Human Growth Hormone (GH) And IGF-1

Also at the Bethesda NIH Conference, Dr. Morris Schambelan of San Francisco General Hospital summarized the results of studies on Serostim GH, with and without IGF-1. The goal of one study was to assess whether a combination approach could reduce the cost of GH therapy. Administration of GH by itself at 6 mg. per day resulted in an average weight gain of 3.2 lbs. after twelve weeks. (Note: 1 mg. of GH equals about 3 IU.) This consisted of a 6.6-lb. lean body mass increase and 3.4 lb fat loss. A quarter dose (1.4 mg. per day) gave a third as much lean body mass increase as the 6 mg. dose. A dose of 1.4 mg. per day of GH plus IGF-1 at 10 mg. per day resulted in a 6.6-lb. lean body mass gain. A dose of 0.7 mg. per day of GH plus IGF-1 at 10 mg. per day resulted in a third of that, at 2.2 lbs. of lean body mass. Another study by Lee of Baylor College in Houston, using .68 mg. of GH per day with 10 mg. per day of IGF-1, showed no net anabolic effect after twelve weeks. Apparently a threshold amount of GH is required for an effect on LBM.

However, whether the LBM gained from the use of GH includes much muscle tissue is controversial. For more details see the section on Growth Hormone in the Anabolic Hormone Guidelines section, Chapter 19.

Anadrol (oxymetholone)

A study published in the *British Journal of Nutrition* showed that oxymetholone, perhaps the most powerful oral anabolic steroid, improved lean muscle mass with what appeared to be no significant side effects in HIV(+) men and women.[58] Oxymetholone, which is sold in the U.S. as Anadrol-50, was given for thirty weeks at a 150 mg. daily dose. Weight gain averaged 14.5 percent of body weight (18 lbs.), which is significant because no controlled exercise program was instituted, and it is known that anabolic steroids exert their greatest effect when weightlifting is employed. Notably, even when patients were burdened with AIDS-related infections, they continued to gain weight on oxymetholone. Caution: 150 mg. is a very high dose of this very powerful steroid.

While oxymetholone is considered to be a powerful steroid with a high potential for side effects, the subjects were reported to have no significant problems with liver function, water retention, virilization, and several side effects thought to be associated with its use. The study didn't look at CD8 T-cell counts, which appear to be more correlative with

survival than CD4 T cells, which were not correlative with weight gain in this study.

We note here that the 150-mg. daily dose is three times what many bodybuilders or powerlifters would use, and thirty weeks is considerably longer than they would generally use this drug. However, our observation is that bodybuilders and powerlifters often combine oxymetholone with other strong steroids, and it may be that this promotes the potential for side effects. Used alone, the potential for problems may be somewhat reduced, especially at lower doses.

ANABOLIC STEROID/AIDS STUDIES NEEDED

While there have been other studies than the few that we have described above, it is clear that a lot more needs to be done in the area of assessing the effect of anabolic steroids on the health and well-being of HIV(+) people. Anabolic steroid use is rapidly becoming part of standard of care as an off-label use. Anabolic steroids, like testosterone and nandrolone decanoate, are among the most economical treatments used in AIDS for their specific purpose.

Reasons for lack of research in this area are numerous: lack of understanding, stigma, and fear of side effects. In addition, studies for unpatentable medicines have a difficult time finding funds. Other problems include the belief that GH, an overly-expensive therapy, which studies show to be less effective than anabolic steroids for lean body mass gains, should be used as the sole compound for wasting reversal; fear that steroids may be immunosuppressive; fear that they induce Kaposi's Sarcoma; fear of abuse; perception from doctors that anabolic steroids are only used for cosmetic purposes; and a belief that they cannot be used by both women and children.

QUESTIONS TO BE ANSWERED

We at PoWeR have written two comprehensive clinical studies with the help of physicians. These studies will evaluate the use of anabolic steroids for lean body mass gains and modulation of immune response. They include nutritional assessment/intervention, anabolic steroids, supervised resistance weight training, immune measurements, and body composition measurements for thirty HIV(+) patients. However, there are many questions that need to be answered in other studies yet to be designed.

Among the many questions that we think should be answered by research studies in this area are:

1. What effect do (higher dose) anabolic steroids have on viral load, if any?

2. What is the most appropriate strategy for application of anabolic steroids to maximize body cell mass gains and minimize any potential long-term effects: maintenance (constant dose, weekly, or biweekly application) or cycling, (escalating/de-escalating dosing plus stacking of two or more compounds which may act synergistically in cycles with a rest period in-between cycles), or a combination of maintenance testosterone with cycled anabolic steroids for periodic increases in growth?

3. What is the best time to intervene to prevent any loss of lean body mass? A study performed in Germany showed that phase angle alpha, one of the variables calculated from BIA, may be one of the best single predictors of survival (better than CD4 T cells) of twelve studied parameters.[69] Phase angle alpha increases with increasing body cell mass. A study designed to show any correlation between anabolic steroid therapy and increases in phase angle alpha might help to answer questions about the chance that anabolic steroids might increase survival in AIDS.

4. What is the effect of body weight above normal Metropolitan Life Insurance recommendations on long-term survival? A cohort study that includes current clinical data from clinical practices around the country could be designed for this purpose.

5. What is the effect of anabolic steroids on CD4s and CD8 subsets at various doses? Dr. Gary Bucher's presentation at the Vancouver AIDS Conference (Abstract Mo.B.423) showed a significant increase in CD8s while using low-dose nandrolone. Our experience with over 3,000 people also shows this effect for a majority of people.

6. What is the effect of anabolic steroids on cytokines like IL-1, IL-6, and tumor necrosis factor? One in-vitro study showed a reduction in IL-1 with testosterone.[70]

7. What is the effect of anabolic steroids on T-cell apoptosis (programmed death of T cells)? An abstract from Germany showed that testosterone decreased apoptosis by 52 percent in an HIV(+) male.[71] This should be looked at to determine if it is beneficial. Is this part of the reason why patients with hypogonadism tend to show decreased survival?[72]

8. What are the best guidelines for females? Drugs like stanozolol, oxandrolone, or methenolone (Primobolan) (not available in the United States) could play a major role in maximizing anabolic effects while minimizing virilization for use by females.

9. What is the best program for pediatrics? Again, oxandrolone or GH used alone, or combinations of oxandrolone and GH, may be an answer to preventing/reversing wasting in this population without stunting their growth.

10. What would happen if we combine cytokine inhibitors like thalidomide with anabolic steroids, especially in patients with active MAC, CMV, diarrhea of unknown origin, or other opportunistic infections?

11. What are the long-term effects of anabolic steroid use on the hypothalamic-pituitary-gonadal axis (HPGA) of HIV(+) people?

12. Is cycling an appropriate way to administer steroids, or should patients be on low doses of anabolic steroids and testosterone continuously?

13. What is the effect of using a high-protein diet and supplements like L-glutamine (shown to be immune enhancing) with anabolic steroid use?

14. What is the effect of using a diet rich in specific fatty acids with anabolic steroid therapy?

15. How effective are the use of Clomid, human chorionic gonadotropin (HCG), and/or anti-aromatases like Arimidex to restore testicular size and testosterone production after anabolic steroid/testosterone therapy? What is the best dosing regime?

16. What are the best guidelines for bedridden patients who are wasting? This population is the one with the most imperative need for treatment and yet is not included in research in this field.

17. What effects do testosterone, other anabolic steroids, and GH have on lipodystrophy, the unusual redistribution of body fat seen in people who are using protease inhibitors?

18. Do anabolic steroids prevent, reduce, or reverse the truncal obesity that is seen in lipodystrophy syndrome?

We believe that studies involving anabolic steroids will deliver more optimal results when they include supervised resistance weight training (or physical therapy for those in the bedridden setting) and controlled high-protein nutrition.

As can be discerned from this list of questions, we are far from answering the basic questions on the optimal use of anabolic steroids for HIV disease therapy. We invite physicians and researchers to join us in this effort.

12

Complementary Approaches Treating Lipodystrophy
by Michael Mooney

While the protease inhibitor (PI) cocktails can bring viral loads down to undetectable levels and have given many HIV(+) people a new lease on life, protease inhibitors are not always benign drugs. As we approach year four of the triple-combo era, numerous problems have appeared among people who are on protease inhibitors. One of the most common of these side effects (and perhaps the least understood) is the "protease belly" or "Crix belly" phenomenon. "Crix belly," so named because it was mostly observed among people being treated with Crixivan, is a condition most notably marked by the appearance of a large protruding potbelly. (At the same time this is happening some people report that they feel like they are losing muscle mass and fat, too, especially in the arms and legs.) Another some-times concurrent but rare condition is the so-called "buffalo hump," which is a fat pad that grows on the back of the neck that resembles what is seen in Cushing's syndrome. Women are also experiencing an increase in breast size as the breasts seem to gain fat (called lipoma), and many people are losing fat in their arms, legs, and cheeks, while one or more of these other things are happening to them. "Lipodystrophy" is the medical term that has been given to this syndrome, but it can also simply be called "bodyfat redistribution."

It now appears that lipodystrophy is not a side effect entirely specific to Crixivan. It may be seen with use of any of the available protease inhibitors, and nucleoside and non-nucleoside analogs. It has also been seen to a lesser degree in HIV(+) people before protease inhibitors were available. However, the various cocktails of powerful drugs being used today to combat HIV seem to increase the severity of this syndrome over the simpler drug combos of a few years ago, although there is discussion that one of the older drugs, D4T (Zerit), may play a central role in the problem (visit http://www.facialwasting.org/pages/891053/index.htm). And in some cases, the addition of the appetite stimulant Megace to the protease inhibitors seems to increase the potential for bodyfat redistribution.

There are several reasons why this might happen. The "protease pouch belly" in many respects resembles the potbelly seen in disease states like Cushing's syndrome, alcoholic hepatitis, and heart disease. In these diseases the potbelly is associated with the development of insulin resistance[73][74][75] and is primarily composed of enlarged fat deposits surrounding the visceral organs, like the stomach, and liver, under the abdominal muscle wall and ribs.[76] The potential for liver burden or toxicity induced by many of the common AIDS medications has been documented, and the protease inhibitors are no exception to this rule. Elevated triglycerides, liver enzymes and blood glucose, and even diabetes have all been observed in patients on protease inhibitor therapy. All of these conditions are symptoms of diminished insulin sensitivity, and we are seeing that the protease inhibitors' effects on liver metabolism are inducing a state of insulin resistance in many people who are on protease inhibitor therapy. Complications of insulin resistance include hyperglycemia (high blood sugar), diabetes, and cardiovascular disease. The FDA has documented over eighty cases of diabetes that appear to be associated with protease inhibitor therapy.

Indeed, from early 1998, numerous studies have documented an association between the use of protease inhibitors and measurements that indicate insulin resistance is present, including data by Kathleen Mulligan, Ph.D., of San Francisco General Hospital, confirming that protease inhibitors can cause the blood chemistry changes that are typical of insulin resistance;[77] Dr. Ravi Walli of Ludwig-Maximilians Universitat Munchen in Germany reporting that peripheral insulin resistance is common in patients on protease inhibitors;[78] and Dr. Andrew Carr of St. Vincent's Hospital of Sydney, Australia, detailing his hypothesis of the cytoplasmic (cellular) retinoic acid-binding protein type I (CRABP-1) biochemistry involved in the liver dysfunction that may promote insulin resistance.[79] Additionally, some people who are using protease inhibitors are being found to have accelerated cardiovascular disease, which is also a common outcome of progressive insulin resistance.

A look at Harrison's *Principles of Internal Medicine* shows us that lipodystrophy can be

Insulin Resistance

Insulin is a hormone that turns on the transport mechanism that brings glucose (sugar energy) into cells to become glycogen. When the cells are resistant to insulin, transport is compromised, so the glucose that cannot be delivered remains in the blood, which results in elevated blood glucose (hyperglycemia). This can lead to increased insulin production by the pancreas as the body increases its effort to transport the glucose, so insulin levels in the blood can increase, too. Insulin is one of the factors that stimulate cholesterol production, so elevated cholesterol can be a direct result of chronically elevated insulin levels. Excess blood glucose can also lead to overproduction of fat molecules (triglycerides), as the glucose is converted to fat for storage.

When there is insulin resistance, distribution of fat molecules in the body generally is dysfunctional. Fat may accumulate preferentially in areas containing the most hormonally responsive fat cells and blood flow, around the internal organs under the stomach muscles and ribs in the visceral cavity (visceral fat).[76] Other areas where there are lots of receptive fat cells with a rich blood supply are behind the neck (brown fat pad) and in women's breasts, and these areas can also be problematic in HIV-related body fat redistribution. Fat may also decrease in subcutaneous fat cells where there are less receptive fat cells with less blood supply,[404] as found in the skin of the arms, legs, and face. A classic example of insulin-resistance associated distribution of fat shows itself in the appearance of a person with a beer gut.

Chronic insulin resistance is associated with diabetes, a distended belly,[76 82] cardiovascular problems, increased risk of cancer,[405-407] and other health problems. Insulin resistance can occur because of liver toxic medications, genetic predisposition, alcoholism, and aging. Consuming too many calories and the intake of excessive amounts of carbohydrates, saturated fats or omega-6 fats (found in common vegetable oils like corn, safflower and sunflower oils) can promote it, too.[109-115]

associated with insulin resistance, and so we see that the components in this puzzle – lipodystrophy, elevated triglycerides, elevated blood glucose, elevated insulin levels; diabetes; cardiovascular disease – are all appearing. While this chapter does not offer a cure for body fat redistribution as protease belly, buffalo hump, loss of facial fat, or lipoma, it offers tools that are documented to improve insulin sensitivity that may help people gain some control over this problem until medical science gains enough of an understanding to solve it.

Does Crixivan Inhibit Testosterone?

Several doctors have told me that they have seen that Crixivan can inhibit testosterone production, and that reduced testosterone production is known to correlate with increased insulin resistance in men.[80]

In contrast, women exhibit insulin resistance when testosterone is elevated.[81] However, reduced testosterone does correlate with increased visceral fat in studies with HIV(–) women.[82] One study showed that about 50 percent of HIV(+) premenopausal women have low testosterone levels, which was associated with low body-cell mass, and a tendency toward having fat mass that is above normal.[83]

It may be that normalizing a testosterone deficiency while being careful about keeping testosterone blood measurements no higher than mid-normal would be beneficial to HIV(+) women to improve nutrient partitioning away from fat tissue while lean tissue increases. This is an area that needs more investigation, as not enough has been done to study testosterone and wasting in HIV(+) women.

We also know that the nucleoside analogs like AZT can cause muscle myopathy,[84] so it can be several things (including low testosterone production) that might add up to a loss of lean body mass and an increase in visceral fat.

While this remains to be proven, one of the things that was presented by Dr. Gorbach from Tufts University when he reviewed their Nutrition for Life Cohort (600 HIV+ men during 254 days on protease inhibitor combos) at the Bethesda National Institutes of Health conference, was that although people tend to put weight back on with protease inhibitors, his data asserts that they regain mostly fat, not lean tissue.

Note: Fat weight is not correlative with survival, but lean tissue is.[85] The loss of lean tissue and reciprocal gaining of fat so that total body weight stays the same is typical of early stage wasting.[86] [87] This increase in fat mass again suggests an impairment in glucose disposal and insulin sensitivity.

For those who have lipodystrophy, I would be concerned about any apparent muscle wasting and have the blood testosterone levels checked, including both free and total testosterone. If total testosterone is low, or in some cases even mid-normal for men, because of the tendency for HIV(+) men to have decreased free testosterone levels, which correlates with a progressive decrease in CD4 T cells,[88] a doctor should consider beginning testosterone replacement therapy. We should also note that free testosterone measurements appear to be more correlative with lean body mass than total testosterone in wasting HIV(+) men[89] and women.[90]

Women and Testosterone

Studies show that HIV(+) women who are losing lean body mass may also need testosterone,[89] but the appropriate dosage of testosterone enanthate injections for women is usually much lower than the dosage for men, between 2.5 and 20 mg. per week. This is something for a doctor to determine by taking blood tests, usually two to three days after the fourth weekly injection for a representative average level. A number of HIV(+) women are using testosterone creams that are compounded by a pharmacy like the Women's International Pharmacy (800-279-5708). However, testosterone enanthate injections deliver a longer-lasting blood level of testosterone than the creams, which have a relatively short lifespan in the body. If a cream is used, it is usually applied in a dose of between 2 and 5 mg. two times per day, while the injections are best given once per week, as studies show that testosterone blood levels generally decline to baseline within about ten days after injection.[91]

As women are much more sensitive to side effects from testosterone, the physician should monitor a female closely for any virilizing side effects, which include oily skin, acne, peach fuzz, hair loss, and clitoral enlargement, and immediately lower the dose or cease the therapy if these kinds of symptoms start to occur.

Normal Testosterone Levels May Not Be Enough (Men Only)

I should also note that finding the correct testosterone dose for each individual is not always easy, as data from studies by researchers like Dr. Judith Rabkin suggests that being HIV(+) can mean that the normal range for testosterone measurements does not necessarily apply to men. In her study with HIV(+) hypogonadal men, Dr. Rabkin found that the dose of testosterone enanthate needed to be above 200 mg. every two weeks, for good quality of life. The dosage she found to be effective was 400 mg. every two weeks (which I suggest is best given as 200 mg. per week for more consistent blood levels, less peak/trough effect, and reduced potential for side effects). At 400 mg. given every two weeks the men's blood testosterone levels averaged about 1,100 ng./dL one week after the fourth injection (on a scale where the normal range is 300 to 990 ng./dL). In private correspondence Dr. Rabkin said that she is not sure whether 300 mg. every two weeks would yield a satisfactory result or whether the men would respond satisfactorily if their average levels only reached 800 ng./dL. She said that some men did receive benefit at about 700 ng./dL though.[92] Remember, the bottom of the normal scale was 300, so the normal scale did not seem to apply well to these HIV(+) men.

Free Testosterone

We assert that some men's apparent need for testosterone at higher than the standard replacement dose of 100 mg. per week (for HIV[–] hypogonadal men) may be the result of hormonal resistance to testosterone. Hormonal resistance appears to happen with several hormones in HIV pathology. However, studies suggest that the need for higher testosterone doses is most likely caused by elevated sex-hormone binding globulins and lowered free testosterone, which is common in HIV.[88 93] When this is the case, total testosterone measurements do not adequately reflect the person's state of health.

Supplementing testosterone to bring free testosterone levels in the body into an optimal range may be beneficial to hypogonadal men in general, by improving the partitioning of nutrients more toward lean tissue and less toward fat tissue, especially visceral fat.[94] Significant data also suggests that appropriate testosterone supplementation can improve blood lipid chemistry to reduce the potential for cardiovascular disease in men who are deficient.[95]

Testosterone Patches or Creams

We have reports that application of the Testoderm TTS or Androderm testosterone patches directly on the "buffalo hump" appears to shrink it. If this works, testosterone creams or gels might work better as the dose of testosterone can be much greater than in a patch. While a study of adipocyte (fat cell) chemistry does provide a rationale as to why application through the skin might work, application of a cream would not be likely to work to reduce the belly because of the greater distance from the skin through the stomach muscles to the fat cells inside.

Anabolic Steroid Improves Insulin Sensitivity and Glucose Disposal

One study showed that the injectable anabolic steroid nandrolone decanoate (Deca Durabolin) improved glucose disposal and lowered insulin levels when administered at 300 mg. per week, while it did not have any effect at 100 mg.[96] While this injectable beta esterified anabolic steroid may have a beneficial effect on insulin sensitivity, another study found that Deca Durabolin appears to enhance non-insulin-mediated glucose disposal.[97] This study and other studies state that oral 17-alpha alkylated anabolic steroids, such as oxymetholone (Anadrol-50), oxandrolone (Oxan-drin) and stanozolol (Winstrol) promote insulin resistance because of their effect on liver metabolism.[98 99] This raises many important questions about using oral steroids when lipodystrophy is present.

The Paradoxical Effects of Oral Steroids

Oral steroids can decrease triglycerides (fats) because of their effect of increasing post-heparin hepatic triglyceride lipase, which breaks down triglycerides.[100 101] For this reason, oral steroids may help to decrease visceral fat, although they promote insulin resistance, and I have heard reports of each of the oral steroids – stanozolol, oxymetholone and oxandrolone – reducing the "protease belly" in HIV(+) males. Indeed, data from a retrospective study of 700 patients recently released by Dr. Douglas Dieterich gave indication that the use of oral and injectable anabolic steroids may be effective in decreasing the potential for lipodystrophy-associated body habitus changes.[102] More study needs to be done to confirm this trend.

Human Growth Hormone (Serostim)

While the relative ineffectiveness of GH as a muscle-building anabolic hormone is detailed in later sections, GH does appear to have a role in reducing lipodystrophy because of its effect on lipid oxidation (fat burning), as was asserted by a poster presentation, from Dr. Gabriel Torres of New York,

that was presented at the XII International Conference on AIDS in Geneva.[103]

Dr. Torres said that while five patients had partial or total reduction of fat redistribution on 5 and 6 mg. doses of GH (which I assert are overdoses for most people), four of the patients (80 percent) had either elevated glucose, elevated pancreatic enzymes, or carpal tunnel syndrome, so GH at these doses increased the potential for serious health problems. Elevated blood glucose can lead to diabetes and the problems that result, including cardiovascular problems, eye damage, and neuropathy; elevated pancreatic enzymes can lead to pancreatitis; and carpal tunnel syndrome is quite painful and may require surgery.

I suggest that if Serostim GH is implemented, it should be considered that Serono's full-vial dose is an overdose, and this may be why 5 and 6 mg. doses caused these problems. It is advisable to adjust the dose down for each individual, in an attempt to gain the benefit without increasing the problems. At this time I have reports of a reduction of protease belly and other types of lipodystrophy with doses as low as 1 mg. per day and up to 3 mg. per day with no side effects. I assert that lower daily doses are safer than higher doses administered every few days, and that at a correct dose, growth hormone can be an important part of the tools that address the underlying metabolic problem. While growth hormone will have a less powerful effect at a lower dose, at the proper individual dose there will still be a significant effect on fat cell metabolism with significantly less potential for side effects.

Exercise

Exercise, too, improves insulin sensitivity,[104] so people with insulin resistance should consider some kind of regular exercise, especially weight training, which also builds lean body mass. Aerobic exercise does not build significant lean body mass. Aerobics may be useful in an effort to reduce lipodystrophy, but if a person is losing lean body mass it should be avoided, at least until the person has regained any lost weight or stabilized. Aerobics will use energy that the body would normally use for rebuilding lean body mass, only accelerating the loss of lean body mass. If your weight is stable and you are not in danger of losing weight, to optimally burn fat and reduce lipodystrophy I suggest doing aerobics three times per week on alternate days to weight training days, first thing in the morning on an empty stomach. (See Chapter 25.)

NUTRITIONAL CONSIDERATIONS

Carbohydrates

I would also suggest altering your diet so that it is balanced somewhat like what might be called an "evolutionary-type hunter-gatherer diet." This means getting more protein and a moderate amount of the healthy types of fats, while eating fewer high-calorie, starchy, complex carbohydrates or high-glycemic, sugary, simple carbohydrates.

Currently, many progressive nutritionists are recommending that people with insulin resistance consider reducing their total calorie intake and intake of high-calorie complex carbohydrates that can release into the blood stream quickly,[105] including wheat breads and most processed wheat products. These kinds of carbohydrates actually are quite calorie dense and can upset insulin metabolism as much as sweets.[106] [107] They are even more problematic when included in high fat foods. (Think pizza and ice cream.) Also on the list of carbohydrates to avoid is the sugar called fructose, which is known to promote insulin resistance, and raise cholesterol.[108] Look for it on ingredient panels as fructose or high-fructose corn syrup. I also underline that some people will experience a reduction in insulin resistance

just by reducing the total calories in their diet, as many people simply eat too many calories. However, if you are having a hard time maintaining weight because of wasting or infection, getting plenty of healthy calories is essential for keeping and building lean body mass, so be careful about reducing your intake of food.

At the same time, I recommend an increase in the intake of complex carbohydrates sources that contain less total calories but lots of fluid and nutrients, like vegetables. Compared to grains, vegetables are more nutrient dense, and less calorie dense. While some vegetables like potatoes and carrots have high glycemic indexes, they supply good amounts of nutrients per calorie, and they do not contain a great amount of calories for their volume like grains or sweets do, so their effect on insulin production, insulin resistance and body fat accumulation is not as great. (Carrots contain only 195 calories per pound, boiled potatoes contain 450 calories per pound, while breads contain about 1,200 to 1,500 calories per pound, and sugar and sweets contain about 1,700 calories per pound.)

Other good carbohydrate sources are beans, yams and green peas, and whole fruits like oranges, grapes, apples, pears, and cherries. In other words try to eat natural food carbohydrate sources that are one step away from nature.

If you do want to include grains in your diet, barley, cream of rye, oatmeal and brown rice have relatively lower glycemic indexes than most wheat products, but be careful to moderate the total amount of these high calorie starch sources. If you include them in your diet, I suggest eating servings that are about one third as much you'd really like to eat. (Again, try to moderate your total carbohydrate calories if your goal is to reduce insulin resistance.)

While a high-carbohydrate diet has been recommended by some nutritionists for conditions of insulin resistance (diabetes), a study by Chen of Stanford University showed that a lower-fat, higher-carbohydrate diet led to higher day-long blood glucose, insulin, and triglycerides, as well as post-prandial (after a meal) accumulation of triglycerides, and increased VLDLs (very low density lipoproteins),[109] which can increase the risk of cardiovascular disease. The idea that lower carbohydrates diets are superior is supported in an article in *Nutrition Reviews* by dietitian Nancy Sheard, who said, "Recent studies indicate that a diet high in monounsaturated fat and low in carbohydrate can produce a more desirable plasma glucose, lipid, and insulin profile."[110] A study published in the *Journal of the American Medical Association* further supported this approach when it showed significantly elevated triglycerides and LDL cholesterol levels with a high carbohydrate diet, while a high-monounsaturated fat diet let to a lower-risk lipid profile.[111]

Fats

While it is also best to reduce any excessive intake of fats, I don't advocate a very low-fat diet, but a reduction in excess saturated fats – found in animal fat products like butter and lard – and excess omega-6 fats, which are found in common vegetable oils, like corn, safflower, and sunflower oils. Excess saturated fats and omega-6 fats can promote insulin resistance.[115] [112] [113] [114] At the same time I recommend a moderate intake of fresh food sources of the essential fatty acid called omega-3, which can reduce insulin resistance,[115] and reduce the potential for atherosclerosis and heart attacks.[116] [117] Omega-3 fats are found abundantly in cold water fish like salmon, sardines, tuna, rainbow trout, anchovies, and herring, and in lesser amounts in flax seed oil, some nuts and seeds and beans, like walnuts, pumpkin seeds and soy beans, and in much smaller quantities in dark green leafy vegetables. Consider also including some daily consumption of monounsaturated fats from sources like olive oil. These too reduce the risk of cardiovascular disease.

Data also suggests that high-saturated fat in the diet promotes more bodyfat accumulation compared to polyunsaturated fats like omega-3 fats.[118] [119] So if you want to be lean, eat clean.

Finally, avoid eating any food that contains artificial fats or processed fats, like hydrogenated or partially hydrogenated oils. Partially hydrogenated oils are found in foods like margarine, french fries, potato chips, shortening, many baked goods, and mayonnaise. Harvard researchers have found a very strong link between these types of unhealthy fats and cardiovascular disease.[120]

Protein

HIV has protein malnutrition as a common theme; a lack of optimal protein contributes to the loss of lean body mass and the trouble of maintaining it. To reduce the loss of lean body mass and to increase it, I suggest that your diet include extra protein that totals at least 3/4 gram per pound of body weight per day. If you lift weights, studies of HIV(–) subjects by world-renowned protein scientist Dr. Peter Lemon show that you may need a total of at least 0.8 grams of protein per pound of body weight per day for optimal increases in lean body mass.[121] [122] If you are not allergic to dairy protein, consider eating cottage cheese as a "best" protein for building muscle, as it contains a great amount of the amino acid L-glutamine, which is discussed below. (Note: Dairy allergy can cause diarrhea.)

Also, consider supplementing your food protein with a protein powder drink two or three times per day. Note that the dairy protein called "casein," seen on labels as "calcium caseinate," appears to have the potential to be somewhat more effective for improving lean body mass than other proteins, like whey.[123]

The Zone Diet

Although I do not agree with some of his more dogmatic concepts, my recommendations for nutrition have some similarities to the "Zone" diet outlined in the book *Mastering the Zone* by Dr. Barry Sears. While aspects of the Zone diet can be criticized scientifically, I have had numerous reports that its use has helped people with HIV reduce cholesterol, the potbelly, triglycerides, and lipodystrophy symptoms, in general.

The Atkins Diet

The Atkins diet is a very low carbohydrate, high protein, high fat diet that can decrease bodyfat significantly. I have reports of people successfully using the Atkins diet to reduce lipodystrophy symptoms. Consider that it is basically impossible to get the RDA of vitamins, minerals or fiber from this diet, so if you use it, take strong multivitamins and extra fiber, and consider that it shouldn't be used long-term. Also, be sure to favor monounsaturated and omega-3 fats over omega-6 and saturated fats.

Dietary Supplements

Supplements that have been shown to improve insulin sensitivity include chromium,[124] and I recommend 200 to 400 micrograms (mcg.) of chromium three times per day in the polynicotinate or picolinate form, as one recent (non-HIV) study showed that 1,000 mcg. of chromium per day increased insulin sensitivity by about 40 percent without toxicity.[125]

The herb silymarin (milk thistle) as a standardized extract in a dose of 200 mg. three times per day has been shown to be effective in improving liver function and improving insulin sensitivity.[126] There has been talk that silymarin can alter liver function in a way that might affect the metabolism of protease inhibitors, so it is possible that people who are taking protease inhibitors should not take silymarin. There is no conclusive data on this yet.

But the best supplement for improving insulin sensitivity and glucose disposal may be the antioxidant called alpha lipoic acid (ALA), at 100 to 300 mg. three times per day.[127] In diabetic studies ALA improves insulin dependent and non-insulin dependent glucose uptake, and it has been shown to effectively lower blood sugar comparable to insulin itself.[128] I believe this is one very important reason ALA is a must for anyone taking HIV medications, especially protease inhibitors. HIV-nutrition expert Lark Lands, Ph.D., asserts that ALA is a must for people with HIV because of its effect on improving glutathione production and recycling.[129] Recent studies at Stanford University showed that glutathione levels directly correlated with increased survival for people with HIV.[130]

As noted by the late Canadian protein chemist Chester Myers, Ph.D., N-acetyl cysteine (NAC) can be a valuable addition to the supplements that address lipodystrophy, because of its effect on improving glutathione, which is necessary for glucose metabolism. I suggest 500 to 1,000 mg. of NAC three times per day.

Also carnitine, as the prescription version called Carnitor, would be beneficial in higher doses, about 500 to 1,000 mg. three times per day, as it helps to lower triglycerides,[131] which are generally elevated when lipodystrophy is present. Note that the acetyl-L-carnitine form of carnitine may be more effective than plain carnitine, but it is more expensive.

Also worth considering is the omega-3 dietary supplement called EPA (fish oil), which has been shown to reduce insulin resistance,[115] and lower triglycerides somewhat in a study with HIV(+) men.[132]

And, taking a strong multivitamin, multimineral supplement that includes chromium, vitamins A, D, E and calcium and magnesium will help improve insulin sensitivity.[133 134 135 136 137 138] I recommend taking a supplement that contains doses that are much higher than the RDAs, as numerous studies have shown that higher nutrient levels are required in HIV disease.[139 140]

Finally, high dose biotin supplementation is frequently prescribed by nutritionally-oriented medical doctors to improve glucose metabolism in diabetes.[141] [142] High dose biotin is also known to improve diabetic neuropathy.[143] The dose of biotin that is commonly used is 1,000 mcg. three times per day.

Cardiovascular Disease

As I mentioned in the beginning of this article, we are also beginning to see cardiovascular disease in people on protease inhibitors. When cardiovascular disease is a consideration, we want to make sure that specific preventive nutrients are included. While there are many that can be included for this purpose, to keep it simple I suggest the following: vitamin E at 400 to 800 IU three times per day to reduce the potential for oxidation of blood fats that can contribute to atherosclerosis;[144] vitamin C at 1,000 to 2,000 mg. three times per day to assist vitamin E in reducing blood fat oxidation;[145] folic acid at 800 mcg. three times per day to reduce the potential for elevated homocysteine, which appears to be another major contributory factor to cardiovascular disease.[146] [147] It should also be noted that vitamins B6 at 50 mg. three times per day and vitamin B12 at 100 to 500 mcg. three times per day help to reduce homocysteine. Of course, all HIV(+) people should consider taking high doses of supplemental B vitamins, as studies by Dr. Marianna Baum of the University of Miami showed that HIV(+) people frequently require six to twenty-five times the RDA of these essential nutrients to stay healthy.[139] [140]

Glutamine

For any loss of muscle, Judy Shabert, M.D., M.P.H., R.D., asserts that supplementing with high doses of the amino acid L-glutamine will help reduce the catabolic process of breaking down muscle tissue,[148] and a recent study of wasting-HIV patients by Prang showed that this might be true. (See Dr. Shabert's article in the August 1997 issue of *POZ* magazine.) For acute wasting, HIV(+) people are using between 12 and 36 grams per day of L-glutamine. (One tablespoon is 12 grams.) I have friends who have halted their random diarrhea and improved their lean body mass using these kinds of L-glutamine doses, and in Prang's study wasting and diarrhea and were checked by using 30 to 40 grams of glutamine per day. Glutamine, too, has been shown to have a powerful effect on improving glutathione production,[149] and glutamine improves insulin sensitivity.[150] [151]

If you are losing weight I suggest that you supplement your diet with a tablespoon of L-glutamine added to each serving of supplemental protein two or three times per day between meals. If your weight is stable, L-glutamine may be supplemented at lower doses, such as one or more teaspoons per day.

Important Note: Most dietary supplements only stay in the blood for a few hours, so it is wise to take them several times per day.

Metformin (Glucophage)

While taking dietary supplements, especially alpha lipoic acid, may help, it is wise to investigate the use of the drugs that are prescribed to improve insulin sensitivity. Ask your doctor about these drugs, which include metformin.[152] New data presented by Saint-Marc at the 6th Retrovirus Conference in February 1999 indicates that metformin may decrease visceral fat while decreasing blood glucose, insulin, and lipid levels.[102] Serostim can increase blood glucose, insulin and insulin resistance.[153] [154] This means that metformin might be found to be superior to Serostim growth hormone because it not only addresses fat redistribution, but reduces some of the underlying metabolic problems that growth hormone can promote. An important consideration is that while 6 mg. per day of Serostim is priced at about $6,000 per month, which makes it inaccessible for a majority of people who have lipodystrophy, metformin is available with a doctor's prescription at any pharmacy, and if people have to pay for it themselves it costs only about $35 dollars per month. However, cautions about the use of metformin are warranted. Dr. Michael Dube of the University of Southern California at Los Angeles states: "Lactic acidosis is a rare side effect of metformin that is more likely to occur when there is some impairment of kidney function. Lactic acidosis, which can be fatal, is also a rare side effect of use of nucleoside analogs. There is no way to know at this time if using the two together might result in more frequent, or more severe, lactic acidosis problems. In my opinion anyway, metformin and NRTI's therefore should only be used together with great caution. Also, keep in mind that metformin can lower vitamin B_{12} levels."

I should also note that some people are finding that switching antivirals causes a marked reduction in some lipodystrophy symptoms. This is an area that is currently receiving a considerable amount of study.

My special thanks go to Jim Brockman, who was the first researcher in AIDS medicine to hypothesize that insulin resistance was involved in bodyfat redistribution. His guidance sparked my investigation into this important area.

The original version of this article appeared in: *Medibolics* 2(2), Nov. 1997. Used with permission.

Addendum, November 2002, Rosiglitazone (Avandia)

New studies show that rosiglitazone, another insulin-sensitizing drug, may benefit those who have lipodystrophy, and may even have some effect on reversing fat loss without some of the problems associated with metformin.[155] Ask your doctor about rosiglitazone. For a valuable and simple brochure on lipodystrophy, visit: http://www.vhconcepts.com/pdfs/2002.changes.pdf

13
Mitochrondrial Damage
by Brad L. Lichtenstein, N.D.

The topic of mitochondrial damage is gaining more and more press as a potential side effect of anti-HIV medication. Simply put, the mitochondria are the "energy factories" of the cell – the tiny, rod-shaped structures, or "organelles," within each cell responsible for producing roughly 90 percent of all the energy that cell needs in order to survive. The number of mitochondria in a particular cell is based upon the energy needs of that cell and can range from 200 to 2,000.

About 80 percent of the energy generated by mitochondria is created through a cellular aerobic (meaning "requiring oxygen") process called oxidative phosphorylation, which creates adenosine triphosphate, or ATP. Creating ATP includes an intricate series of steps that involve five multi-sub-unit enzymes or complexes. Each complex has a different nutritional and chemical need in order to function properly. This is important to remember when exploring the nature of treatment for mitochondrial damage.

As mitochondria produce ATP, they simultaneously yield reactive oxygen species (ROS), which are harmful free radicals that circulate throughout the cell, the mitochondria, and the body, causing more damage. The circulation of ROS leads to the activation of reactive nitrogen compounds, which in turn induce, or activate, genes in the DNA that are associated with many degenerative diseases such as

Alzheimer's, Parkinson's, strokes, and multiple sclerosis. The term "mitochondrial toxicity," therefore, is a misnomer and actually refers to the process of mitochondrial damage.

The DNA for each mitochondrion (mtDNA) remains unprotected within the membrane of the mitochondrion itself. In comparison to the DNA in the nucleus of the cell (nDNA), mtDNA is easily damaged by free radicals and the ROS that they produce. Freely floating mtDNA lacks protective measures associated with nDNA, and therefore mtDNA suffers from multiple mutations.

It has been estimated that this lack of protective measures results in mutations to mtDNA occurring 10 to 20 times more frequently than mutations to nDNA. The mitochondria that are produced have decreased ability to function, resulting in the inability to utilize fatty acids for energy production, and therefore a decreased ability to store fat in muscle tissue.

In order for mitochondria to reproduce themselves, a specific enzyme called gamma-DNA-polymerase, or "pol gamma" is required. Many medications have been found to interrupt pol gamma. Studies suggest that virtually all the nucleoside analog reverse transcriptase inhibitors (NARTIs) – such as AZT, 3TC, ddI, ddC, d4T, and abacavir – interrupt pol gamma to some extent. This disruption prevents the transport of long-chain fatty acids from being transported through the membrane wall into the mitochondria, where they are used as primary fuel and energy sources. As a result, fatty acids are dysfunctionally deposited and accumulated in muscle tissue. Without the cell's main source of energy, the number of newly formed mitochondria drops, and therefore, cell function decreases, and possibly even cells die (or apoptosis). Symptoms developed by an individual would depend upon the type of cell affected. However, the most common symptom is generalized, overall fatigue.

Test tube (in vitro) studies have demonstrated that ddC, ddI, and d4T are the most potent inhibitors of pol gamma, although the other NARTIs exert some influence as well. To date, researchers have not studied the extent of mitochondrial damage when anti-HIV medications are combined, which is standard practice for most individuals currently on anti-HIV therapy. Moreover, the effect of combining NARTIs with other anti-HIV medications, such as protease inhibitors, is not known.

However, one study demonstrated a reduction in the number of mitochondria produced in a cell in people taking d4T. Data from yet another small study suggested that HIV(+) individuals taking any of the NARTIs had up to 44 percent fewer mitochondria per cell than those individuals who are either not taking NARTIs or are HIV(–). One study demonstrated that those taking AZT had significant depletion of mitochondrial DNA in muscle tissue.

In a study examining the number of mitochondria per cell, participants were separated into four groups: (1) HIV(+) individuals who were on medications and had fat loss/wasting, (2) HIV(+) individuals on medications without signs of fat redistribution, (3) HIV(+) individuals who had not taken anti-HIV drugs and (4) individuals who were HIV(–). The group with the greatest decrease in mitochondria in cells was the group with fat loss/wasting, followed by the HIV(+) group on medications yet without signs of lipodystrophy. The latter two groups showed no

difference in number of mitochondria. The conclusion drawn is that anti-HIV medications do interfere with production and lifecycle of mitochondria.

It has been postulated that mitochondrial damage is always present, but the question is to what extent. Mitochondrial damage is poorly diagnosed, and when symptoms do occur, they can run the range from mild, to severe, to life threatening. For instance, common symptoms include fatigue, muscle weakness (myopathy), peripheral neuropathy, and pancreatitis. However, some researchers suggest that regardless of HIV serostatus, damage to mitochondria can be a possible factor in low platelet count (thrombocytopenia), anemia, and low neutrophil count (neutropenia). Furthermore, there is a significant link between damaged and dysfunctional mitochondria and the development of Type II diabetes in adults, again, regardless of HIV serostatus.

With early enough detection, many of these symptoms and conditions are reversible by altering therapy. This may include stopping medication, or significantly reducing dose. However, people considering such a course of action should first consult with their healthcare provider to identify the specific cause for the symptom.

How can mitochondrial damage be detected? The easiest way is through a blood test that measures lactate levels in the blood. Lactate is a natural byproduct from the breakdown of glucose and fat in the mitochondria. The sore and tired feeling in the muscles following rigorous exercise is a result of the body shifting to "anaerobic respiration" that leads to a buildup of lactic acid. When the mitochondria are damaged, lactate levels rise in the bloodstream and lead to lactic acidosis. This increase in the acidity in the blood is life threatening and must be dealt with immediately. Lactic acid level in the blood should be measured (without a tourniquet, if possible) after a person has been resting for at least 5 minutes, and has refrained from vigorous activity and alcohol consumption for 24 hours.

Early symptoms of lactic acidosis are severe fatigue, nausea, vomiting, shortness of breath, abdominal pain, rapid weight loss, muscle cramps and aches, muscle numbness and tingling, and rapid and progressive muscle weakness. As the severity increases and lactate levels rise over 5 mmol/liter (the normal value is less than 2), mitochondria lose their ability to produce energy, leading to potentially irreversible organ damage and death.

At present, there are no comprehensive studies presenting clear treatment strategies for dealing with mitochondrial damage associated with HIV. Extrapolation can, however, be made from the knowledge available about treatment of mitochondrial damage associated with other diseases. First and foremost is to identify and treat the cause. For many, however, this option may be limited. If it is true that the main associated factors are the NARTIs, then switching to another therapy might be suggested. Eliminating this entire class of HIV medication from treatment options leads to a whole host of medical and health-related issues. It does seem, at this time, that ddI, ddC, and d4T are the most potent inhibitors of pol gamma. This should be considered for those suffering from mitochondrial damage. The availability of Viread (tenofovir) has provided a good alternative to other NRTIs for many people. Viread does not appear to affect mitochondrial function.

Finally, several nutrients have been studied for their ability to decrease damage to the mitochondria. In the current literature regarding mitochondrial damage and HIV therapies, some mention has been made about carnitine, coenzyme Q10, and riboflavin (B2). Most of these are being studied in isolation and not in conjunction with one another. Although the approach is to determine whether or not each particular nutrient is beneficial in the treatment of mitochondrial damage, the flaw in this approach stems from the fact that each of the five complexes in the oxidative phosphorylation process requires different and varying nutrients simultaneously. Other nutrients that support mitochondrial function are alpha lipoic acid, NAC (N-acetyl-cysteine), vitamin E, and essential fatty acids, to name a few.

Carnitine is a natural substance found in food, mainly meat and dairy products, that can be quickly absorbed in the small intestines. The standard daily American diet contains roughly between 10 to 100 milligrams of carnitine. The body can synthesize carnitine from the essential amino acid, lysine, with vitamin C, niacin, vitamin B6, iron, and the amino acid methionine as necessary cofactors. Carnitine is vital to the life of the cell since it is required for the transport of long-chain fatty acids into the mitochondria. Regarding supplementation, two forms of carnitine have been used, either L-carnitine or acetyl carnitine. Studies show that supplementation with L-carnitine decreases the percentage of both CD4 and CD8 cells undergoing cell death (apoptosis.)

Furthermore, supplementation with L-carnitine has been successfully used in the treatment of mitochondria-induced muscle weakness and degeneration. Studies with patients taking AZT reveal low levels of carnitine found in their muscle tissues. Several studies explored the use of 6 grams of L-carnitine daily intravenously. The results revealed a reduction in serum triglyceride levels, an increase in peripheral blood mononuclear cell-associated cermainde (an intercellular messenger of apoptosis), and a decrease in tumor necrosis factor (a cytokine that is produced as a result of infection, which intensifies viral replication). Another study, in which HIV(+) patients with severe neuropathy were given daily intramuscular injections of 1 gram of acetyl-carnitine (the form of carnitine more easily absorbed in the intestines), showed decrease in patient report of pain and improved movement and mobility. Overall, carnitine is necessary to keep mitochondria alive and functioning well, thereby resulting in the proper nerve and muscle function, fatty-acid synthesis, and energy production.

No RDA (recommended daily allowance) has been established for carnitine. Studies range in the amounts used for mitochondrial and neurological benefits. No side effects have been reported, but this author has had patients report slight gastrointestinal pain within a half-hour of taking carnitine orally. Current trends recommend between 1,000 to 4,000 mg. of L-carnitine or acetyl carnitine in divided doses daily. Because carnitine is an amino acid, it is best absorbed on an empty stomach.

Carnitine works synergistically with another nutrient, the fat-soluble vitamin-like compound called coenzyme Q10 (CoQ10), also known as ubiquinone. CoQ10 is an essential factor in the electron transport chain, the pathway from which ATP and metabolic energy is derived, which occurs within the mitochondria. CoQ10 is a strong antioxidant that resides in the lipid membrane surrounding the mitochondria and protects it against free-radical damage. Although the body can generate its own CoQ10, supplementation has been shown to be warranted in persons with HIV. CoQ10 is synthesized in the cells of every living organism in nature. The body produces CoQ10 in a 17-step process that requires riboflavin (B2), niacinamide (B3), pantothenic acid (B5), pyridoxine (B6), cobalamine (B12), folic acid, vitamin C, and other trace minerals. Due to its complex and intricate requirements, nutritional deficiencies with any one of these vitamins can disrupt mitochondrial energy production. Generally, symptoms of CoQ10 deficiency affect cardiovascular health in the form of congestive heart failure, stroke, arrhythmias, high blood pressure, mitral valve prolapse, and cardiomyopathy. Additionally, lack of energy, gingivitis, and overall weakened immunity are symptoms of CoQ10 deficiency.

Many medications directly deplete the body of CoQ10. While antiretrovirals have not been studied for their effect on CoQ10 levels, both antiretrovirals and antibiotics, such as Bactrim and Dapson, deplete the body of the B-vitamin family. Other medications, specifically cholesterol-lowering medications, anti-hypertensive medications like beta-blockers, and some tricyclic antidepressants like amitriptyline (at times used for treatment of neuropathy) all directly deplete the body of CoQ10, and thereby negatively impact the mitochondria. The studies of HIV-positive individuals who are either on antiretroviral medications or are drug naive reveal CoQ10 deficiencies.

Supplementation with CoQ10 has shown decreased incidence of opportunistic infections and improved immune parameters, measured by a reduction in symptoms such as night sweats, fever, diarrhea, weight loss, and lymphadenopathy.

Again, no RDA has been established for CoQ10; yet, current recommendations range from 30 to 120 mg. per day, depending upon the severity of symptoms and health status. No side effects have been reported for CoQ10.

Riboflavin or B2, is a water-soluble vitamin, that, like other B vitamins, is not stored well in the body so must be ingested daily. Riboflavin belongs to a category of yellow colored pigments called flavins (the reason urine changes color when taking B vitamin supplements). When riboflavin interacts with phosphoric acid it becomes a part of two essential enzymes. These enzymes are necessary for the conversion of carbohydrates to energy in the form of ATP within the mitochondria of the cell. Furthermore, deficiencies in riboflavin will exacerbate CoQ10 deficiencies. For these reasons, riboflavin supplementation has been considered in the treatment of mitochondrial damage. Many medications, such as antiretrovirals, antibiotics, oral contraceptives and the tricyclic antidepressant noritriptiyline result in direct riboflavin deficiencies. No major studies have demonstrated a direct improvement in mitochondrial health with supplement of riboflavin. However, since multiple cofactors are required in energy production in the mitochondria, studies of riboflavin alone may be misguided.

Typical symptoms of frank riboflavin deficiencies are inflamed mucous membranes, chelosis (cracks in the corners of the mouth), soreness and burning of lips, tongue, and mouth, burning, itching and tearing eyes, eczema of skin and genitals, light sensitivity, dry and itching scalp, nerve damage, depression and hysteria.

The recommended daily allowance (RDA) for riboflavin is approximately 1.7 mg. per day. For pregnant women, nursing mothers and heavy exercisers, higher doses are recommended. Several studies have used dosages in the range of 2 to 100 mg. per day.

Several other nutrients, which are beneficial to the health of the mitochondria and immune system, need mention here. The first, alpha lipoic acid, is a powerful antioxidant. Alpha lipoic acid is found in highest concentration within the mitochondria, and helps protect against damage to the cell's membranes. In vitro, alpha lipoic acid has been demonstrated to inhibit tumor necrosis factor, NF-kappa B, the on-off switch for activation of HIV, and tat gene activity. In Europe, alpha lipoic acid has been used successfully for the treatment of diabetic neuropathy, leading to its study in the efficacy of treatment for HIV-related neuropathy either as a result of medication or the virus itself. Because of its ability to cross the blood brain barrier, alpha lipoic acid has been recommended as a potential treatment for cognitive disorders as well. Alpha lipoic acid has been shown to heal liver cells, decrease elevated liver enzymes, and lower high blood glucose. An added benefit of alpha lipoic acid is its ability to recycle vitamin C and vitamin E, and to increase blood levels of glutathione. No RDA exists for alpha lipoic acid, but use ranges between 100 to 1,200 mg. per day. However, one study postulated that high doses (above 1,200 mg. daily) may result in thrombocytopenia, decrease in platelet counts, but this has not been replicated. Standard practice often recommends 200 mg. twice a day.

One of the most significant benefits of N-acetylcysteine (NAC), the sulfur-containing amino acid, is its reported ability to raise glutathione levels. Glutathione is the primary antioxidant system within the body, thus aiding the body against free radical damage. While the literature is still unclear as to whether or not supplementation with oral glutathione will in fact raise tissue stores of glutathione, the majority of studies do conclude that NAC supplementation will raise glutathione levels. Many medications and substances deplete glutathione, such as acetaminophen, sulphamethoxazole (Bactrim), and alcohol, and protease inhibitors deplete liver stores of glutathione, thus the recommendation that those with HIV infection refrain from using large amounts of acetaminophen.

Additionally, NAC supplementation leads to a "relative" increase in CD4 cells and a reduction in HIV-1 replication in stimulated CD4 cells. Dosage suggestions vary considerably with ranges between 1,000 mg. to 8,000 mg. per day having been studied. Side effects of higher dosages include gastrointestinal distress that can be alleviated by taking NAC with food. Standard protocols suggest between 1,000 mg. and 3,000 mg. per day in divided doses.

Finally, dietary fat has a major impact on the health of mitochondria. Trans-fatty acids, fat sources from hydrogenated and partially hydrogenated vegetable oils, directly affect the membranes through which fats must be shuttled to be used by the mitochondria for energy. The greater the amounts of trans-fatty acids in the diet, the less fluid can easily pass through. As mentioned earlier, the production of ATP involves five multi-subunit complexes. Studies suggest that trans-fatty acids might inhibit ATP production by inhibiting complex V in the process. Therefore, diets high in saturated fats and trans-fatty acids are to be avoided in order to prevent damage to or improve the function of mitochondria. Rather, essential fatty acids such as flaxseed oil and fish oils should be recommended to ensure healthy membranes surrounding mitochondria.

Mitochondria are sensitive organelles whose function and health can be easily disrupted. In searching for "treatments" for mitochondrial damage, many researches continually focus on one nutrient or one substance to restore balance. Since the ATP system is complex and requires a large number of nutrients, such a singular search will often fail to yield a significant result. For this reason, a series or group of nutrients needs to be explored. L-carnitine (acetyl-carnitine), CoQ10, and B vitamins would be an excellent starting point for someone suffering with mitochondrial damage. Since all nutrients have multiple bene-

fits, those interested in expanding their protocol should consult about any supplementation program with a qualified healthcare provider well versed in HIV medications as well as diet and nutrition.

Brad S. Lichtenstein, N.D. is a licensed naturopathic physician, personal trainer, and yoga and meditation teacher. In private practice, he specializes in HIV care, counseling, and yoga therapy. This article was provided by the Seattle Treatment Education Project. *STEP Perspective*, Volume 02, Number 2, Fall 2002. Visit their web site at http://www.thebody.com/step/stepix.html   Used with permission.

For a comprehensive supplement that includes all ingredients needed for mitochondrial protection, visit the Houston Buyers Club website and look for the "Metabolic Protective Formula," http://www.houstonbuyersclub.com/ (800-350-2392).

14
HIV-Related Facial Wasting:
Potential Reconstructive Procedures
by Nelson Vergel

For more information, visit www.facialwasting.org and join lipodystrophy@yahoo groups.com by sending an email to: Lipodystrophysubscribe@yahoogroups.com

Facial wasting is currently one of the most important issues in the lives of those living with HIV. A person's HIV status sometimes becomes apparent just by looking at his or her face. Self-image and self-esteem issues are now arising because of this. A poster presentation was given at the second International Workshop on Adverse Drug Reactions and Lipodystrophy in HIV (LIPO 2000 Conference) in Toronto, September 12-15, 2000. It dealt with, "Erosion of self-image and self-esteem; problems in society and threats to locus control; anxiety around HIV disclosure forced by noticeable body change; and a propensity to demoralization and depression." (Collins, Abstract P36).

Some HIV(+) people have reduced or minimized visceral fat growth ("protease belly") with the use of nutrition, exercise, anabolic therapies, insulin sensitizers and switching HIV medications. However, facial wasting and the loss of subcutaneous (under the skin) fat are problems that have seen no consistent solution. Some studies that have followed patients after they switch from protease inhibitors to non-nucleoside analogs have not found statistically significant changes in body composition. However, a study presented by Saint Marc, et al., and the Retrovirus Conference in February 2000 found that the loss of subcutaneous fat could be reversed partially by switching from Zerit (Stavudine or D4T) to Abacavir (Ziagen) or Combivir combinations. Dr. Andrew Clark from South Africa also presented a poster (Abstract P85) that showed improvements on facial wasting after switching from Zerit to an alternative NRTI antiviral in ten of eleven patients after six months. After talking to investigators, all concur that although these studies show a potential reversal of this problem, the fat gains in the facial area are very slow and still not sufficient to bring the original look back to someone's face. (For more on Zerit and fat loss, visit http://www.medibolics.com/Lipoatro-phy andAntiretroviralDrugChanges.htm and http://www.hivandhepatitis.com/hiv_and_aids/lipo/lipo8a.html)

Out of despair and necessity, many HIV(+) people are searching for reconstructive techniques that could improve their facial wasting. Cosmetic techniques like Bio-Alcamid (polyalkylimide gel), collagen injections, Fascian, Alloderm, silicone injections, New Fill, polymethyl methacrylate (PMMA) and polyacrylamide gel and others are currently being used by many people who have had to cash life insurance policies to pay for these procedures because they are generally not covered by insurance.

Where Are Implants Placed?

Traditionally, skin is divided into three layers, epidermis, dermis and hipodermis. The epidermis is composed mainly of cells, while the dermis contains extracellular matrix, nerves, vasculature, and adnexal structures.

Injectable soft tissue fillers generally are injected into the dermal layer. The dermal layer allows for host incorporation of the material due to the presence of fibroblasts in the extracellular matrix and vasculature. Fibroblasts help encapsulate the material to keep it in place. Some materials preferably are placed in the subcutaneous layer due to implant nodularity and palpability, i.e., the way it "feels."

If you have experienced side effects and harm from an implant, if you believe a physician may not be following IDE requirements, or if you believe that a physician is charging excessive amounts of money for an IDE-based procedure (over "cost recovering" amounts), write a complaint letter to:

Dr. Larry Kessler
Center for Devices and Radiological Health
Food and Drug Administration
Office of Surveillance and Biometrics (HFZ-70)
9200 Corporate Boulevard
Rockville, MD 20850

Investigational Device Exemption (IDE) Protocols
Approval of Implants in the US

From http://www.fda.gov/cdrh/devadvice/ide/index.shtml

IDE Overview

An investigational device exemption (IDE) allows the investigational device to be used in a clinical study in order to collect safety and effectiveness data required to support a Premarket Approval (PMA) application or a Premarket Notification [510(k)] submission to FDA. Clinical studies are most often conducted to support a PMA. Only a small percentage of 510(k)'s require clinical data to support the application. Investigational use also includes clinical evaluation of certain modifications or new intended uses of legally marketed devices. All clinical evaluations of investigational devices, unless exempt, must have an approved IDE before the study is initiated.

Clinical evaluation of devices that have not been cleared for marketing requires:

• an IDE approved by an institutional review board (IRB). If the study involves a significant risk device, the IDE must also be approved by FDA;

• informed consent from all patients;

• labeling for investigational use only

• monitoring of the study and;

• required records and reports.

An approved IDE permits a device to be shipped lawfully for the purpose of conducting investigations of the device without complying with other requirements of the Food, Drug, and Cosmetic Act (Act) that would apply to devices in commercial distribution. Sponsors need not submit a PMA or Premarket Notification 510(k), register their establishment, or list the device while the device is under investigation. Sponsors of IDE's are also exempt from the Quality System (QS) Regulation except for the requirements for design control.

Options For Facial Lipoatrophy

1. **Fat grafting:** Fat is liposuctioned from one area of the body and then injected into the areas of concavity in the face. This requires a relatively modest surgical procedure to "harvest" fat. Some of the harvested fat is injected at that time, and the rest is frozen to use as needed on subsequent office visits. Comment: Some patients may not have sufficient fat that can be transferred to the face. Furthermore, the transferred fat seems to be absorbed quickly by the body, so additional procedures are required. General anesthesia and an overnight hospital stay are required. A presentation at the 2002 Third European Conference on Lipodystrophy and Metabolic Disorders (ECLMS) in Marbella, Spain (April 2002) showed that most of the transferred fat is reabsorbed after nine months.

2. **Facelift:** Surgical lifting and tightening of the skin can achieve quite dramatic results. A facelift is a complicated surgical procedure and generally requires a longer period of healing than other techniques available for correction of facial concavities.

3. **Dermal/fat grafts:** This technique requires placing a piece of the person's own skin with attached underlying fat into the area of facial concavity in order to restore fullness. In the experience of several plastic surgeons, this procedure gives the longest lasting and most natural results. General anesthesia and a hospital stay are required, and the fat grafts may disappear in a few months.

4. **Artificial filling materials:** A variety of different materials are manufactured which can replace a person's own fat. These materials include Collagen, Dermalogen, Fibrel, Goretex and others. Some of these materials have a more lasting effect than others. Additionally, however, these materials are more antigenic than a person's own tissue and may have a higher incidence of infection and other complications.

For the last twenty years, methods for filling facial wrinkles and crevices have been flourishing in the field of cosmetic treatment. Each method has its advantages and disadvantages. Until the present time, two broad categories of implant have been available to the physician:

- **Biodegradable implants** (of animal or biological origin), usually of animal origin, the therapeutic effects of which are limited in time (rapid resorption by the body). This category notably includes collagen (of bovine origin; allergic reactions are possible in 2 or 3 percent of patients) and hyaluronic acid (very rapid resorption).

- **Collagen suspensions** have been widely used over the last decade. The results have been found to be generally disappointing since collagen is absorbed by the body in one to three months. Allergic reactions are also observed in approximately 2 percent of patients. Lastly, it should be noted that the collagen is of bovine origin.

- **Hyaluronate gels** provides a good alternative due to their biocompatibility and absence of toxicity. They are, in fact, widely used in eye surgery, but their rapid resorption by the body (two months at most) makes them unsatisfactory for plastic surgery.

- **Biological material taken from the patient**. While this idea was certainly an interesting one, clinical experience has since shown that implantation of the patient's own fat cells is ineffective, due to the fact that they are absorbed and disappear in a matter of weeks. Another solution would be to add the patient's plasma to a collagen gelatin of bovine or porcine origin. The results of this are even more disappointing. In addition, this material is of animal origin.

- **Synthetic, non-biodegradable implants**, whose long-term effects are uncertain. Examples: liquid silicone (a base material banned in France, which leads to local and systemic complications that are well known), and PMMA, HEMA or EMA microspheres (acrylic base material: Plexiglas). Silicone is banned in most countries. While infection is always a possibility with use of any of these materials, some materials have unique complications. Silicone can cause foreign body reactions and rejection of the implant for up to twenty years following implantation. Synthetic implants of any kind can produce nodularity if placed in an improper plane. The risk for developing granulomas and migration can be present even after ten years. We have no long-term safety data of any synthetic implant product used in HIV(+) people.

- **Silicone gel (or silicone oil):** Silicone injection into facial tissues was popularized in the 1960s and 1970s with the introduction of medical grade silicone (MDX 4-4011) by Dow Corning. Microdroplets of silicone are dispersed within the dermal tissues. Fibrosis around these droplets localizes the material, and it is seemingly well tolerated in small amounts in the face. Silicone oil has many advocates among those who used it prior to Food and Drug Administration (FDA) withdrawal of approval. However, silicone, although chemically well tolerated,

becomes encapsulated as a foreign body by a chronic inflammatory reaction. Giant cells surround the material and cannot process any ingested material, establishing a low-grade inflammatory nidus. Fibrous tissue surrounds and encapsulates the silicone; this capsule is avascular and is a potential site of infection. A number of late infections, granulomas, and palpable masses have been reported following silicone use. It has been observed following injections that silicone droplets migrate into the tissues under the injection site, simply drawn there by gravity. Silicone is a frequent cause of granuloma and even of delayed allergic response. Silicone is not biodegradable and is often detected in the human liver.

Silicone injections have been used for many years in the gay community in big cities. Female impersonators have used it to alter their faces, buttocks, and breasts. Non-medical personnel have performed the procedure in people's homes. No known reports of severe reactions have been reported due to the illegal and underground nature of this procedure. Many people living with HIV have obtained silicone injections in the past through non-medical personnel in Miami, Los Angeles, and New York.

The FDA has not approved the marketing of liquid silicone for injection for any cosmetic purpose, including the treatment of facial defects or wrinkles, or enlarging the breasts. The adverse effects of liquid silicone injections have included movement of the silicone to other parts of the body, inflammation and discoloration of surrounding tissues and the formation of granulomas (nodules of granulated, inflamed tissue). However, there is a protocol, currently in the design phase, for the use of silicone micro-droplets (SilSkin). This may be a safer method. For more information about this protocol, email anna@carruthers.net (Dr. Carruthers is in Vancouver, Canada, and there are four centers in the U.S. and one in Canada.) For more information about the product and research sites, email drichard@richard-james.com, and/or visit Dr. Derek Jones's website at www.derek jones.com, or Dr. Orentriech's (New York City) website at http://www.orentreich.com

Some U.S. physicians are currently using a silicone product, called "Silikon 1000," off label, for facial wasting. This product is FDA approved ONLY for use as a long-term tamponade for complex retinal detachments, but can be used legally "off-label" for facial lipoatrophy.

- **The SoftForm facial implant** is a persistent yet removable facial implant for the treatment of deep facial furrows or creases such as nasolabial folds (creases between the nose and corners of the mouth), deep frown lines and definition of the vermilion border surrounding the lips. The implant will provide a substantial correction of the furrow or creases. However, it may be necessary to use another product such as Collagen Replacement Therapy® to achieve full correction of the treatment area. The SoftForm facial implant is a hollow, tube-shaped implant made of a biocompatible polymer called ePTFE (expanded polytetrafluoroethylene). The ePTFE polymer is a proven material which has been used for more than twenty years in a variety of medical applications that include the replacement of deteriorating blood vessels in over 3.5 million people, hernia repair, abdominal wall reinforcement and, subsequently, for soft tissue augmen-

tatation of the face. This procedure is not widely used for facial wasting.

- **Teflon® paste** consists of a suspension in glycerin of particles of polytetrafluoroethylene (particle diameter 10 µ to 100 µ). This material has led in many cases to severe chronic infections and it has proved necessary to remove it from the dermal and subdermal tissue of most patients after a few months. It has also been demonstrated that small polytetrafluoroethylene particles can be detected in the liver.

- **Bioplastics** are polymerized silicone particles (diameter 70 µ to 140 µ) dispersed in polyvinylpolypyrrolidone. It proved necessary to withdraw this material from the market completely due to the chronic inflammation and rejection responses it caused.

- **Microspheres** of polymethylmethacrylate (PMMA), hydroxyethylmethacrylate (HEMA) and ethylmethacrylate (EMA), with diameters in the ranges 20 µ to 40 µ or 40 to 60 µ, placed in a gelatin suspension or solution, a collagen solution or a hyaluronate gel. HEMA and EMA are not used as much anymore. PMMA has ten years of research in humans. In addition, in some cases the vector used is once again a collagen of bovine origin (in Brazil, the vehicle used is hydroxyethylcellulose, a cellulose [plant fiber] solution). The desired material is an implant allowing controlled resorption. The aim would be first to find a type of implant offering a resorption period of one year in order to allow possible cosmetic adjustments. PMMA has been used successfully by Dr. Marcio Serra in Rio de Janeiro, Brazil (email: mserra@dermatologista.net or mserra@netfly.com.br) in over 220 HIV(+) patients for over three years. The cost for the entire procedure in Brazil is $500 (two sessions needed). Dr Serra does the implants in the subcutaneous (sub-dermal) area to avoid granuloma formation. No long-term safety data is available. The trademark in Canada (and soon in the U.S.) for PMMA is Artecoll. Another PMMA product is Metrex. Anecdotal reports from patients who obtained one session of Artecoll in Canada are not very encouraging. (Artecoll may need more than one session.) After an interview with Dr. Gottfried Lemperle, one of the researchers of Artecoll, I was informed that some doctors are very conservative about injecting too much Artecoll at a time since it cannot be removed after its application, so one session is not enough is most cases.

- **Polylactic acid (New-Fill),** also called PLA (http://www.new-fill.com/Page/Anglais) is a biocompatible, bioabsorbable synthetic polymer belonging to the family of aliphatic polyesters. Its safety is an acknowledged reality, as is shown by the toxicology studies and a range of medical and surgical applications over a number of years (rheumatology, reconstructive traumatology). Its bioabsorbability is well established, and its resorption is controllable, verifiable, open to modulation to satisfy various criteria, and reproducible. For most people it takes three to five sessions for moderate facial wasting, and six to seven sessions for severe facial wasting. Touch ups are needed after a year. Approximate cost of each session is $600 to $800, which includes the product, so the total cost without travel expenses can be anywhere from $1800 to $5600. For a list of

U.S. doctors using this product, go to: http://www.thebody.com/tpan/septoct_ 01/new_fill.html (Prices on this website are no longer valid.)

- **Polyalkylimide gel (Bio-Alcamid):** This product has been used in Italy for six years as a gel type prosthesis in plastic surgery without major complications. I started hearing about it at the beginning of 2001 from people in Los Angeles and San Diego, who were reporting good results and durable effects with only one to three sessions, so I decided to investigate it. Everyone had gone to Clinic'estetica in Tijuana to get the procedure done by Anna Love, who has nine years experience and has trained cosmetic surgeons from the United States. A presentation at the ECLMS conference in Marbella, Spain (April 2002) made by Dr. Jose Arevalo showed good and lasting results in over 100 patients during the past three years. One to two sessions were needed to correct most cases. No "touch ups" are needed unless lipoatrophy continues. It seems that two of the advantages of Bio-Alcamid is that it can be removed easily if too much product is injected, and large quantities can be injected (ideal for buttocks also) without a significant immune response. The manufacturer sent me an email to ensure that I did not confuse this product with polyacrylamide gel since they believe polyalkylimide is much more stable than polyacrylamide gel (there have been reports of bacterial contamination of polyacrylamide gels from Russia). Presently, the only source of this product in North America is Anna Love at http://www.clinicestetica.com/. The average price for full facial restoration is $4500. You also have to consider your travel expenses to Tijuana (two or three trips). Pictures of different applications (implants in different body parts like buttocks, face, chin, nose, biceps, etc.) can be found in the Italian website: http://www.bioalcamid.com/index2.htm

Conclusion

The impact of facial lipoatrophy on self-image and self-esteem is devastating for the HIV surviving community. Several non-FDA approved options for lipoatrophy related facial reconstruction are emerging to deal with this problem that may be induced by HIV medications. Patients can access these products in Mexico, France, Brazil or through FDA-approved IDE protocols in the U.S. In all instances, including U.S. protocols, the patient has to pay amounts that exceed $3,000. No reimbursement is currently available for these options. Furthermore, no long-term data is available, so it is difficult to assess safety of any of these options. Current information is limited to small studies with no clinical data besides before-and-after pictures. Some options may require frequent touch ups and others tend to be more permanent. A comprehensive and effective advocacy campaign is needed from the HIV community to lobby to the FDA for all important issues, for safe protocols and for access for those who may want to make an informed decision based on risks and benefits. Additional advocacy in the area of reimbursement is also needed since these are corrective measures that treat a drug-induced side effect. Like any other side-effect corrective measures that are available, it should be reimbursable by third party payers. Hopefully, we will see progress on this issue in the near future.

Please address any comments or concerns to me at powertx@aol.com. The author and facialwasting.org do not assume any responsibility for the decision a person makes after reading this information. This information is to be shared with your physician for further discussion. All of these procedures lack long-term safety data in HIV(+) patients.

15

Testosterone and Anabolic Steroids: Adverse Effects, Rumors and Reality

by Michael Mooney

There is considerable misunderstanding on the part of the public and the medical community regarding the true potential for adverse effects that may occur as a result of the use of testosterone and anabolic steroids. This holds true both for legitimate medical reasons at appropriate conservative doses and for non-medical (cosmetic or athletic) uses at high doses. I assert that analysis of all of the available data will yield a more balanced perspective that will position anabolic steroids as being clearly less dangerous than most of the medications that are commonly used for HIV therapy, including protease inhibitors, antiretrovirals, antifungals, and many other drugs. I have heard doctors and other people express concern that anabolic steroids can cause cardiovascular problems, cancer, prostate problems, immune suppression, Kaposi's sarcoma, lymphoma, and other health problems. Some cautions are warranted, but the potential for these health problems is sometimes exaggerated, and in some cases, non-existent.

Indeed, none of the several dozen studies on anabolic steroids and HIV(+) subjects have documented a significant association with any specific health problem so far. And with thousands of HIV(+) subjects using anabolic steroids since 1982, anecdotal evidence suggests that if anabolic steroids used in medically appropriate doses are causing significant health problems they are somewhat rare. Also note that steroids may cause subtle problems, like sleep apnea, that have not yet been clearly documented in HIV(+) subjects, which may define themselves as time goes by.

Cardiovascular Disease

While there are many questions about adverse effects, one of the most common areas of misunderstanding centers around the idea that all anabolic steroids increase the risk of cardiovascular disease. Certain steroids, like testosterone, nandrolone and oxymetholone have more potential to promote increased blood pressure, which will promote cardiovascular problems if not effectively addressed. However, while many people assume that all steroids cause the blood lipid changes that promote cardiovascular disease, there is a considerable difference in the minimal effect on lipids that can be caused by oil-based injectable beta-esterified steroids, like testosterone enanthate and testosterone cypionate; the generally non-existent or small effect caused by nandrolone, another beta-esterified steroid; and the pronounced effect caused by the oral 17-alpha alkylated steroids. Oral steroids have had profound effects on lipids, seen in elevated LDL cholesterol, and decreased HDL cholesterol that may increase cardiovascular risk, where nandrolone has much less effect and testosterone has little, if any, significant effect.[156][157][158][159] This is why injectable steroids appear to be a wiser choice if cardiovascular risk is to be reduced.

In fact, good data suggests that appropriate testosterone replacement might reduce the risk of cardiovascular disease. For instance, clinical studies with elderly and hypogonadal men have shown a beneficial effect on blood lipids with testosterone replacement.[160] Recommended reading on this subject includes two books by German physician Jens Moller: *Testosterone Treatment of Cardiovascular Disease – Principle and Clinical Experience* (out of print), and *Cholesterol – Interactions with Testosterone and Cortisol in Cardiovascular Diseases* (ISBN 3-0540-17097-9). Both of these books are Springer-Verlag publications.

Prostate Cancer

Other misunderstandings are related to the idea that testosterone replacement therapy might raise prostate specific antigens (PSAs) or cause prostate cancer. While there is one case study that states that testosterone replacement increased PSA secretion in one man,[161] other larger studies assert that there is no significant effect on PSAs with appropriate testosterone replacement.[162][163] And, while some studies show no association between testosterone and prostrate cancer risk, other studies assert that higher testosterone levels correlate with an increased risk of prostate cancer.[164] Note that low serum testosterone, too, has been described as resulting in a poorer prognosis in advanced prostate cancer.[165] (It may be that too much testosterone increases progression of prostate cancer, but so does too little testosterone.) Still, while most data shows a distinct association between testosterone and tumor growth, a study of 100 prostate cancer patients showed no association between free testosterone, total testosterone, and tumor volume.[166] Other data supports the idea that estrogen dominance has a significant effect on prostate growth, especially with advancing age where testosterone

declines relative to estrogen,[167][168] therefore inhibition of estrogen may be beneficial. This is definitely a complex issue that needs more controlled clinical data to resolve, but prudence dictates that if testosterone replacement is found to be necessary, the lowest effective dose should be used, and any individual with a potential for risk should be followed closely, including monitoring PSA.

Liver Toxicity

The potential for liver toxicity is another misunderstanding that is common with anabolic steroids. Specifically, injectable beta-esterified (oil-based) steroids are not toxic to the liver, while oral 17-alpha alkylated (17AA) steroids present some toxicity to the liver in a dose-dependent manner.[169][170]

However, the potential for acute liver toxicity with 17AA steroids appears to be considerably less than many other medications, with potential problems related to hepatic toxicity, including cholestatic jaundice with short-term use, and with long-term use there have been rare reports of peliosis hepatitis and benign and malignant neoplasms (tumors).[171][172][173][174] To be clear, as detailed by Zimmerman of Georgetown University, 17AA anabolic steroid-induced cholestatic jaundice usually manifests as "bland" cholestatis rather than the more potentially lethal inflammatory cholestasis. In general, neoplasms have occurred only with very high-dose 17AA steroid use (100mg/day) over periods of two to four years, with eleven years as the longest recorded use that resulted in carcinoma.

These side effects are dose and duration dependent, and are two of the reasons that we recommend that the use of oral 17AA steroids be limited to 12-week cycles or the shortest amount of time that is necessary to gain the desired weight. For a reprint of Zimmerman's essay titled, "Hepatic Effects Associated with the Clinical Use of 17A-Alkylated Anabolic-Androgenic Steroids," email a request to access@access-medical.com.

For a comprehensive review of the literature related to testosterone's benefits versus its potential for problems in HIV therapy, I suggest reading a paper by Dr. Judith Rabkin titled, "Testosterone Treatment of Clinical Hypogonadism in Patients with HIV/AIDS," published in the *International Journal of Sexually Transmitted Diseases and AIDS*.[175]

16
Anabolic Hormones:
Adverse Effects and Remedies
by Michael Mooney and Nelson Vergel

Anabolic steroids are medicines with good risk-to-benefit ratios, but they do have the potential to cause side effects, and each of them can produce side effects when the dosage is high enough. Some steroids are less likely to cause problems though, especially when used in their correct dosage window. This is a brief look at possible side effects, with a list of the remedies that might help. Use the prescription items listed below only when monitored by a doctor, as several of them, like Accutane, can be dangerous.

Problem	Solution and Comments
Acne/oily skin – Caused by testosterone and oxymetholone, less by nandrolone, generally not caused by oxandrolone or stanozolol in men, but may cause problems for women.	Accutane – a powerful prescription item – 40 mg./day for one week sometimes stops acne if started at the first sign or as directed by your doctor. Accutane is potentially highly liver toxic. Sporanox – Effective for some acne-like eruptions that are caused by fungi. Some doctors also prescribe antibiotics, like tetracycline, for acne with good results. Anti-bacterial soaps – Use a scrubbing brush and wash twice a day, especially after sweating during a workout. UV light or sunlight with moderation.
Hair loss – Caused by too much testosterone, and by oxymetholone. Rarely seen with nandrolone, oxandrolone or stanozolol, but they may cause problems for women.	Proxiphen salve and NANO shampoo/NANO conditioner – These and other hair loss products are formulated by Dr. Peter Proctor (713-960-1616). Nizoral shampoo – Available by prescription and over-the counter as a lower dose product. Rogaine – Available by prescription. Propecia (finesteride) – Available by prescription. A few males experience decreased erections with finesteride, though. Hair Regrowth Formula (visit www.medibolics.com).

Problem	Solution and Comments
Increased sex drive – Caused by testosterone and oxymetholone more than other steroids.	A problem? Sex drive can decrease in HIV. Sex drive is part of quality of life. This is not necessarily a bad side effect. Enjoy it.
Impotence during a steroid cycle – Rarely caused by testosterone, much more by other steroids. This happens more with steroids other than testosterone because they do not support healthy sexual function in the same way that testosterone does. That is why we recommend that all steroid cycles be built on a testosterone foundation.	Viagra – Available by prescription; enables robust erections. Yohimbine – Available by prescription; increases sex organ sensitivity. Muse – Available by prescription; inserts into the penis to produce erection. Trimix – Available by prescription. The best and cheapest formula for injection into the penis for lasting erections. Visit Visit www.appliedpharmacyrx.com or call 251-478-6768. Caverject – Available by prescription. An injection into the penis that produces an erection that can last 1 to 2 hours. Be careful with injecting too much since it can produce dangerously long erections that need to be treated in emergency rooms! Follow instructions from your urologist. Papaverine – An older injectable medication, less expensive than Caverject. Wellbutrin – Prescription at 300 to 450 mg./day; increases dopamine. Human chorionic gonadatropin (HCG) – First dose is 5,000 IU, then taken again one week later. Note: If impotence happens while on testosterone, try varying the doses of testosterone, e.g., higher and lower. New prescription drugs in the pipeline – Cialis, Uprima. Read medibolics.com for updates!
Insomnia – Usually this is caused by dosages that are too high. Find the least amount that gives you a good result.	Sleeping medications – e.g., Ambien, Sonata, Restoril Melatonin – 1 to 3 mg. before bedtime. Avoid working out too close to bedtime. Limit caffeine, especially after 3 PM. Do not administer oral steroids after 6 PM. Visit www.appliedpharmacyrx.com for a comprehensive sleep formula with tryptophan, melatonin and inositol (prescription needed). Nutrients do not work as well as drugs, but they can help some people.

Problem	Solution and Comments
Sleep Apnea	Have a sleep specialist prescribe a sleep study. Some people may have to wear a C-PAP machine to breathe at night. Visit http://www.sleepapnea.org/ for more information
Testicular atrophy – Caused by all steroids.	HCG – One 5,000 unit injection per week for two weeks.
Enhanced assertiveness – mostly testosterone, and oxymetholone, but they can all increase drive depending on dosage.	Great! HIV(+) individuals often have low energy, so this means wake up and live, or workout harder at the gym. Decrease caffeine. Practice meditation, yoga. The steroid dosage may be too high, especially testosterone and oxymetholone.
High blood pressure/water retention – testosterone, oxymetholone, nandrolone.	Sometimes this is caused by elevated hematocrit or water retention and sometimes by steroid doses that are too high. High blood pressure is associated with chronic use of steroids, though. Blood pressure medications – Elevated blood pressure is usually transient and stops within a few weeks of the end of a steroid cycle. However, ongoing or chronic steroid use is associated with high blood pressure. Try ACE or ACE II inhibitors since they seem to have fewer sexual-dysfunction-related effects. Supplements – Magnesium (600 mg./day); vitamin B_6 (100 to 200 mg./day); may help reduce water retention. Water – Drink extra water every day to help flush the kidneys.
Virilization (body hair growth, deepened voice, clitoral growth in women) – Caused by testosterone, less by oxymetholone and nandrolone, much less by stanozolol. Generally not caused by oxandrolone.	Discontinue steroid use or only use steroids that have the lowest androgenic potential, like oxandrolone. We note that GH used with steroids seems to exacerbate body hair growth in males. Proscar – Available by prescription at 1 to 5 mg./day, for men.

Problem	Solution and Comments
Gynecomastia (male breast development) – Caused by overproduction of estrogen, which can happen when there is too much testosterone. (Testosterone converts into estrogen.) Oxymetholone use is sometimes involved. Nandrolone is less likely to, while oxandrolone and stanozolol shouldn't. Growth hormone can also promote it. See the sections on Growth Hormone in Chapter 19 for more information.	Arimidex – Inhibits estrogen production. Available by prescription. 1 mg./day until sensitivity stops, then 1/2 mg. per day. Nolvadex – Competes with estrogen for receptors. Available by prescription, 10 to 20 mg./day. Not as effective as Arimidex. Use of Nolvadex during a steroid cycle may reduce the net anabolic effect, as it decreases the production of GH[176] and IGF-1. Severe cases may require removal of the breast tissue by surgery. See: http://www.drnadler.com/gynecomastia.htm DHT cream – Some people have obtained great results by rubbing a 10 percent DHT cream on their nipples. Visit www.applied-pharmacyrx.com for more information about this compounded prescription cream.
Prostate enlargement – testosterone and oxymetholone. Nandrolone less. Stanozolol and oxandrolone have even less potential to cause this and may not have an effect at all. This is not clear.	Prostate enlargement – testosterone and oxymetholone. Nandrolone less. Stanozolol and oxandrolone have even less potential to cause this and may not have an effect at all. This is not clear. Proscar – Available by prescription. For men, 1 to 5 mg./day. (Note: Can cause decreased sex drive in some men.) Hytrin – Available by prescription. Saw palmetto extract – Very effective for reducing prostate problems, but one study suggests that this herb may reduce the effects of testosterone, too.[177] Estrogen inhibitors like Arimidex. Estrogen dominance appears to increase prostate growth.[178] [179] Check your prostate specific antigen and have a digital rectal exam before starting any steroid program, to detect potential for prostrate cancer, especially if you are over thirty-five or have a family history of prostate problems, and have it checked on a regular basis.

Problem	**Solution and Comments**
Polycythemia (Elevated hematocrit, which means there are too many red blood cells) – Caused by testosterone, nandrolone and oxymetholone, much more than oxandrolone or stanozolol.	Therapeutic phlebotomy means to have a pint or more of blood removed, usually 1 pint per week over several weeks. (Removing one pint usually will lower hematocrit by about 3 points.) Polycythemia is a compelling reason to avoid using higher steroid doses than are necessary. Taking the lowest effective dose reduces the risk of over-production of hemoglobin (red blood cells).
Elevated liver enzymes – Incidence is often exaggerated, but is related to 17-alpha alkylated oral steroids, not oil-based injectable steroids. Note: Injectable stanozolol, which is not approved for human sales in the U.S., is also 17-alpha alkylated.	Standardized silymarin (milk thistle herb) – 160 mg./three times/day. LiverCare – two 640 mg. tabs twice per day. Evening primrose oil – 1300 mg./three times/day. Lung Tan Xie Gan – Chinese herb formula. Alpha lipoic acid – 100 to 300 mg./three times/day. Glycyrrhizinate Forte – Three or more capsules/day, but this may increase blood pressure. N-acetyl cysteine – 600 mg./three times/day. Glutamine powder – 4 to 12 grams/three times/day. Omega-3 fatty acids – 6 to 10 capsules per day. With a history of liver problems or Hepatitis C, avoid oral steroids and use only injectable steroids – testosterone or nandrolone. Antioxidant vitamins – Vitamin C – 1,000 to 2,000 mg./three times/day with vitamin E – 400 to 800 IU three times/day. Selenium – 200 mcg. twice per day. Alpha lipoic acid – 100 to 300 mg. twice per day. We recommend Jarrow brand slow-release alpha lipoic acid. Visit www.houstonbuyersclub.com for a comprehensive formula for liver health

17

Anabolic Steroids and Kaposi's Syndrome

by Nelson Vergel

Some physicians fear that implementing anabolic steroid therapy may induce Kaposi's sarcoma (KS) or increase its progression. KS has been found to be caused by a herpes-family virus. Although no controlled research has been performed on this, there is data that infers a relationship between hormones and KS. For instance, there is research showing that corticol steroids like prednisone can increase KS progression in HIV(+) patients.[180][181][182] (Note: Corticol steroids are not anabolic steroids, but they are sometimes confused with each other.) Some researchers hypothesize that, since most forms of KS are more common in men than women,[183] there must be a connection between male hormones and KS. Two notable papers on this topic were presented at the 1993 International AIDS Conference (Japan). One investigated whether hormonal factors contribute to a higher incidence of KS in men than women, and found no relationship.[184] The second paper found that men with KS had significantly higher levels of dehydroepiandrosterone (DHEA) and estradiol than those HIV(+) non-KS patients with the same CD4 levels.[185] When compared to non-KS patients, DHEA and testosterone were higher in patients with more than 500 CD4s; DHEA and testosterone were higher in patients with 200 to 500 CD4s, and DHEA was higher and testosterone lower in patients with less than 200 CD4s. It also found that estrogen and glucocorticoids were not significantly different in the two groups.

Notably, this study found that the decrease in CD4 counts and progression to AIDS is accompanied by a decrease in serum testosterone. Unfortunately, other hormones in the hypothalamic-pituitary-gonadal axis that may play a role here, such as leutinizing hormone (LH), and follicle-stimulating hormone (FSH), were not measured in this study.

Another study done on men with CD4s below 132, which did measure total and free testosterone, estrogen, luteinizing and follicle stimulating hormones, found that all patients with KS had lower testosterone and estrogen levels, and higher FSH than KS-free AIDS patients, AIDS-related complex patients, and asymptomatic HIV(+) individuals.[186] A study performed in women found that low estrogen is common in females with KS, HIV(+) or not.[187] So, there appear to be confusing patterns with high/low testosterone or estrogen levels. It may be that another hormonal factor is involved, maybe something women's bodies produce that makes them less susceptible to KS than men. I think part of the answer to this question may be found in the studies that are looking at the beta form of human chorionic gonadotropin (b-HCG) as a treatment for KS. Women produce HCG during the early stages of pregnancy and it is extracted from their urine. One study showed that KS cells are killed in vitro and in vivo (apparently by apoptosis, programmed cell death) by b-HCG.[188] Dr. Robert Gallo observes that women's KS lesions subside during pregnancy.[189] He notes that b-HCG is similar to leutinizing hormone, which is produced at high levels during the menstrual cycle. This, he says, may account for the observation that KS occurs less in HIV(+) women than men. He does not point at men's higher testosterone as a culprit for this difference in incidence.

Many doctors have success injecting b-HCG in KS lesions. Notably, HCG increases men's testosterone production dramatically. So, HCG may help treat KS, but at the same time it increases testosterone. (This is another weak link in the theory that testosterone increases KS.) Dr. Marcus Conant (San Francisco), Dr. Parkesh Gill (USC-LA), Dr. Walter Jekot (Los Angeles), Dr. Patricia Salvato (Houston), and Dr. Gary Bucher (Chicago), assert that they haven't seen a higher KS incidence in patients being treated with anabolic steroids. Furthermore, Dr. Bucher concluded a 73-patient study using nandrolone decanoate. Eight of them had KS prior to the study. At conclusion, no significant differences in KS were seen between the controls and participants. Dr. Bucher feels sure that there is no anabolic steroid/KS relationship.

The incidence of KS has dropped dramatically with the advent of protease inhibitors. I have seen dozens of people go into remission once they start protease inhibitor therapy.

We welcome a clear resolution to this question through controlled studies, but at this time it appears that there is no direct relationship between testosterone and KS. Since KS is less common, this may not be as relevant as it once was.

18

Anabolic Steroids for AIDS Therapy
A Comparison Table
by Michael Mooney

The table that follows, on pages 77-78, is designed to clear up some of the misconceptions regarding anabolic steroids as therapeutic agents for AIDS-related wasting therapy. This table is a guide to weighing the relative risks-to-benefits for some of the common steroid analogs that are available in the United States and other countries. It merges anecdotal information from my survey of doctors and athletes over many years and the published data. All anabolic steroids can inhibit the body's production of its own testosterone, and all can produce side effects when the dose is high enough.

Notes About the Comparison Table

Five stars = highest rating; one star = lowest rating. Some good muscle-building steroids are given lower ratings because they may have more potential for side effects.

1. Nandrolone decanoate (Deca Durabolin) and testosterone are paid for by insurance for many people. If your pharmacist cannot obtain nandrolone, have him or her call Watson Pharmaceuticals. If you have to pay for it yourself, Applied Pharmacy Services (formerly Gulf-South) honors prescriptions for nandrolone for about $125 per 10 cc vial containing 200 mg. per cc. Applied Pharmacy also supplies injectable testosterone for one of the lowest prices in the United States, and oxandrolone at $385 for sixty

12.5 mg. capsules. This is much less inexpensive than the normal price of about $1500. Call: 877-729-1015, or go www.appliedpharmacyrx.com

2. Some studies show that specific anabolic steroids have beneficial effects on specific immune functions.[190] [191] [192] [193] [194] Differences in how specific anabolic steroids affect the immune system in HIV should be studied. Many AIDS doctors prescribe testosterone and the other anabolic steroids and see improvements in critical components of the immune system, such as CD8 T cells.[194] Studies show that testosterone can delay the progression of immune diseases, like the autoimmune disease lupus.[195]

3. Common oral/tableted steroids are 17-alpha alkylated. This presents a burden to the liver that can cause an increase in liver-specific blood tests because they may be somewhat toxic to the liver in a dose-dependent manner. When Hepatitis C is present, do not use oral steroids; use only injectable oil-based steroids, such as testosterone or nandrolone. Do not use oral steroids when taking Atazanavir. Injectable steroids (except injectable stanozolol, which is 17-alpha alkylated and not sold in the U.S.) do not cause any significant liver burden.[196] [197] Injectable steroids are generally preferred over oral steroids for this reason. However, injectable steroids may appear to cause elevations in multi-purpose liver function

tests (SGOT/AST, SGPT/ALT, and LDH) during increased muscular stress or other stress in the body. Steroid-free athletes with high metabolic and muscular stress may show some elevation of some of these blood tests, too. Numerous other drugs also elevate these blood tests. Liver test elevations usually reverse with cessation of the steroids. Anecdotal evidence from competitive bodybuilders who use steroids in high doses, and published data in the medical literature suggests that the incidence of liver toxicity from oral steroids is somewhat exaggerated and rarely creates severe problems in healthy humans. I suggest that physicians be particularly sensitive to the discrete liver readings – bilirubin, GGT, and the liver isoenzyme of LDH. Data suggests that these are more consistent indicators than the multipurpose liver tests, like SGOT/AST and SGPT/ALT, when looking for potential liver problems related to anabolic steroids.[198] [199] Of course, it is prudent to respond to all aberrant liver function tests when drug metabolism is complicated with compounds like the standard AIDS medications or Hepatitis C.

"Virilizing" means masculinizing. This can mean increased body hair growth, a deeper voice, etc. in males and females. Women may find that they start to get oily skin and acne, grow dark peach fuzz or a mustache or other body hair, have itching of the clitoris followed by increasing clitoral size, or develop other male characteristics with continued administration of steroids that are somewhat androgenic. These problems sometimes reverse if the steroid dose is not too high and steroid use is stopped immediately when side effects are detected.

4. "Anabolic" refers to the growth of muscle and is desirable for wasting therapy. Optimal lean body mass is highly correlative with survival in AIDS.[200] While increased androgenic potential can mean more potential for side effects and virilizing, some androgenic potential is necessary for healthy metabolism as natural androgenic activity is necessary for libido, energy, and healthy brain chemistry. Generally speaking, the less androgenic a steroid is, the less side effects there will be. However, all anabolic steroids have some androgenic potential, and steroids that have very low androgenic potential usually have less anabolic potential.

5. The upper dosage listed for women is usually for severe wasting only. Women's bodies do not tolerate anabolic steroids as well as men's bodies do, in general, so doctors agree that it is best to be conservative in the dosages, except in special circumstances where there is severe wasting. The steroids that are more androgenic, like testosterone, may not be problematic if the dosage is appropriately low. It is wise to consider starting at the lowest dosage possible when women use androgens/steroids.

Disclaimer

Dosages listed are based on a survey of the dosages used by medical doctors, and are not the author's suggestions. This information is for your doctor's evaluation and is not to be construed as information to be used for self-medication. If you self-medicate, you do so at your own risk, as no responsibility is implied or intended on the part of the author or the publisher. These dosages are somewhat conservative and only provide a reference range; actual patient needs are highly individual. The dosage ranges given in this table have been verified by medical doctors familiar with AIDS therapy to generally cause no significant side effects when used appropriately.[201 202 203]

Comparison of Anabolic Steroids

Steriod	Anabolic	Androgenic	Effects and Side Effects with Reported Effective Dosages
Testosterone Enanthate or Cypionate ✪✪✪✪ (Injection) Required for most steroid cycles. Available in U.S. and other countries. Very inexpensive.	High	Medium to high	For HIV(+) men, 100-200 mg. per week for maintenance, strong effect on libido, energy, appetite. Higher doses increase potential for water retention, hair loss, acne, gynecomastia (breast growth), mood changes and polycythemia. Supports immune function.
Nandrolone Decanoate ✪✪✪✪ Trade name: Deca Durabolin (injections) Best steroid for men. Available in U.S. and other countries. Inexpensive.	High	Low to medium	Very good lean muscle growth. For men, 100-400 mg. per week is relatively safe for three-month anabolic cycles. A twelve week NIH-funded men's HIV study used 600 mg. per week. Can cause some water retention and polychythemia. May decrease libido if used without testosterone. For women, 25 mg. per week up to 50 mg. for severe wasting only. (There is a chance of virilization).
Stanozolol ✪✪✪+ Trade name: Winstrol (oral) Available in U.S. and other countries. Good steroid for men. Can be used by women. Relatively inexpensive oral steroid. (80 cents per 2 mg. tablet = 40 cents per mg.)	Medium	Low	For men, 6-18 mg. per day added to 100-200 mg. per week of testosterone. For women, may use 4-8 mg. per day, with slight chance of virilizing. No water retention, but watch liver enzymes. (See note 3.) Seems to increase the effectiveness of other steroids when used in combinations.
Stanozolol ✪✪✪+ Trade name: Winstrol (injection) Not available in the U.S. Included here because some HIV(+) people obtain from overseas and self-administer.	Medium	Low	For men, 50 mg., 3 times per week. For women, 15 mg., 3 times per week. No water retention, but watch liver enzymes as this water-based injectable steroid is 17-alpha alkylated. Slight chance of virilizing for women.

Steriod	Anabolic	Androgenic	Effects and Side Effects with Reported Effective Dosages
Oxymetholone ✪✪✪✪ Trade name – Anadrol-50 (oral) Available in the U.S. and other countries. Strongest oral steroid; 50 mg. per tablet. Least expensive oral steroid per milligram. ($12 per 50 mg. tablet = 24 cents per mg.)	Very high	Medium to high	For men, 10-100 mg. per day. Most powerful, least costly oral steroid for building muscle. Can support libido. Dose-related potential for hair loss, increased blood pressure, water retention, body hair growth, gynecomastia, etc. HIV study with males and females, at 150 mg. per day for 30 wks., showed no significant side effects, and 14 percent weight gain. (I am skeptical of the lack of side effects.) Some women are reportedly using 25 mg. per day without problems. May decrease liver glutathione production. Watch liver enzymes.
Oxandrolone ✪✪✪ Trade name: Oxandrin (oral) Good steroid for women and children. Some men get good results, some do not. Results can be very good when used with testosterone. Available in U.S. and other countries. Expensive ($5.35 per 2.5 mg. tablet = $2.14 per mg.)	Low to medium	Very low	For women, 5-15 mg. per day. For children, 1/10th mg. per kg. of body-weight or 2.5 mg. per day. Does not stunt growth in children. For men, 20 mg. or more per day added to 100-200 mg. per week of testosterone. Possible liver toxicity at doses above 20 mg. per day for adults. May interact with the P450 3A4 enzymes that metabolize protease inhibitors.

Program for Wellness Restoration (PoWeR) Anabolic Hormone Guidelines

by Michael Mooney and Nelson Vergel

Introduction

Testosterone and androgenic-anabolic steroids are rapidly becoming common therapies in the treatment of HIV disease for males and females who experience loss of lean body mass or hormonal deficiencies. These compounds have been used since the early 1980s by progressive doctors in Los Angeles for HIV wasting therapy and are now being used by many more doctors around the country. Dr. Walter Jekot, the first doctor to discover that androgenic-anabolic steroids were beneficial for AIDS therapy, in the early 1980s, had patients who were using testosterone or anabolic steroids for cosmetic bodybuilding purposes when they came down with the new disease that was later to be called AIDS. Dr. Jekot noticed that his patients who used steroids maintained higher T-cell counts and suffered from fewer opportunistic infections than his patients who were not using steroids, who progressed more rapidly and died. This is how Dr. Jekot discovered that anabolic steroids were beneficial for AIDS patients. After much initial skepticism, we found a number of inferences in the medical literature that support Dr. Jekot's contention that steroids, like testosterone and nandrolone, may actually support healthy immune metabolism and improve long-term survival in HIV.[204] [205] [206] [207] [208] [209] [210] We have also interviewed some of Dr. Jekot's long-term patients and their statements support his position.

Recently released results of several controlled studies show the safety and efficacy of the use of these steroid hormones for HIV therapy. With the publication of these studies and the information that is available about the most effective methods for administration, there is little reason for HIV(+) people to experience wasting.

Our directive is to gather and refine information about anabolic hormones provided by doctors, the bodybuilding community, and HIV(+) individuals themselves, and share it with other HIV(+) people and their doctors. To date there have been over 100 studies in the U.S. and around the world that have investigating therapeutic anabolic hormone use for HIV. We have assisted some of these researchers to ensure that these studies include information already known by bodybuilders and the doctors who have worked with them. Anabolic steroids have been available since the 1950s and there is an abundance of non-HIV related information available to facilitate current research in this area. These documents summarize guidelines we have designed that are in use by clinicians across the country to treat HIV-related wasting and improve body composition for optimal health and longevity for HIV(+) individuals.

Rationale

There are several reasons for the administration of steroids:

1. When the person's body does not produce adequate amounts of testosterone or free testosterone, the use of continuous testosterone replacement supports optimal physical and mental health and quality of life.

2. When a person has lost lean body mass, testosterone, combined with anabolic steroids, promotes rapid gain in lean body mass. Use of this kind of combination is generally only necessary for a period of several months.

3. Maintaining lean body mass and a feeling of well being over the long-term for some people requires testosterone replacement combined with a low dose of an additional anabolic steroid.

4. As part of a comprehensive program to address lipodystrophy.

Testosterone Replacement Therapy

Many male[211] and female[212] HIV(+) individuals do not have adequate testosterone function, primarily because the body's natural testosterone production is impaired, the amount of bioavailable testosterone is reduced, or there is inadequate expression of testosterone's effects at the cellular level. These may be complications of HIV-infection, but there may be other lesser known reasons for hormonal dysfunction, like nutrient deficiencies that impair production of hormones or their reception and expression, e.g. zinc, vitamin A, and potassium deficiencies can decrease testosterone production or utilization.[213 214 215]

With progression of HIV, hormonal changes have significant correlations with immune function. Studies show that hypogonadism in HIV(+) people significantly correlates not only with loss of lean body mass,[211 212] but also decreasing T-cell count[212] and increasing morbidity.[216] One recent study suggested that testosterone replacement therapy might decrease apoptosis (programmed T cell death) in HIV(+) hypogonadal males.[217]

In another study with HIV(+) men, DHEA and free testosterone levels decreased as CD4 T cells decreased in all patients.[218] In this study, low levels of free testosterone were common in all HIV and AIDS patients, and total testosterone and androstenedione were lower in those patients whose CD4 T cells were below 200.

For those who are deficient in testosterone, replacement therapy should be implemented using doses that are tailored for each individual. Once the appropriate dose is determined, the person will generally experience improved quality of life, including better appetite, energy, improved mood, healthy libido, and immune function, and improvements in weight gain, functional strength and physical hardiness, while suffering no significant side effects.

It appears that most HIV(+) people who need testosterone therapy will have to use it at replacement levels for the rest of their lives, or until a cure is found.

The Antidepressive Effect of Testosterone

We frequently hear HIV(+) people tell of how testosterone replacement therapy ended a long-time feeling of depression. One comparative study stated that testosterone replacement therapy produces equivalent effects to common antidepressive drugs (imipramine, fluoxetine, and sertraline) in the treatment of clinical depression in HIV(+) people.[219] While testosterone is not specifically defined as an antidepressive agent, restoring testosterone levels in hypogonadal patients can produce a powerful antidepressive effect, possibly via its effects on neurological systems (dopamine),[220] and dramatically improve feelings of quality of life. Testosterone also has a very important effect on enhancing healthy libido for men and women.[221 222] Dr. Judith Rabkin is now conducting a study to compare testosterone to Prozac.

Measurements

All HIV(+) people should be evaluated for testosterone function at HIV diagnosis and several times per year thereafter, first to see if they are producing enough testosterone, and then to see if they are responding optimally to the testosterone that their body manufactures by questioning them about energy, libido, mood, appetite, etc. Many HIV(+) people appear to be hormonally resistant to testosterone and do not respond adequately to what are considered to be normal blood levels of testosterone, so the doctor should consider that some people may require higher doses to experience testosterone's benefits.

Inadequate testosterone function means either that the person is documented to have low free testosterone blood levels, low total testosterone levels, or they do not respond normally to testosterone levels that measure in the normal range.

Hormonal resistance can express itself as low libido, low energy, decreased appetite, depression, decreased immune function, loss of body weight, decreased muscle tissue or functional strength.

It appears that a majority of male hypogonadism in HIV is caused by pituitary dysfunction, rather than testes problems.[211] To determine if the problem is in the brain or the testes, the physician should test for luteinizing hormone; if there is relatively normal or elevated luteinizing hormone coming from the brain, but low testosterone production coming from the testes, the problem is in the testes' ability to respond to luteinizing hormone. In HIV, testes problems can be caused by a number of factors including cytokine-induced inhibition of leydig cell function.

Hormone blood tests should be performed before any use of testosterone or steroid cycles. These include free and total testosterone for males and females to determine baseline measurements so that the doctor has complete information about the patient.

Elevated Hematocrit

Before any use of testosterone or anabolic steroids we also advise that the doctor measure hematocrit, as testosterone and anabolic steroids can increase hematocrit significantly, especially when higher anabolic doses are used. Thereafter, hematocrit should be monitored quarterly during any use of testosterone or anabolic steroids. We are also seeing an unusual increase in hematocrit when anabolic steroids are used with some of the protease inhibitors, especially Crixivan, so this may be an unusual effect of this combination that should be taken into consideration.

Some people will experience elevated hematocrit and hemoglobin with the use of testosterone injections, GH, or some anabolic steroids, which can increase the risk of strokes. If these are required for the person's quality of life and overall health, we suggest that the physician consider that these elevations can be addressed by the administration of therapeutic phlebotomy (removal of one pint of blood) rather than interrupting the use of these hormones. Phlebotomy of one pint of blood will generally lower hematocrit by about 3 percent. We have seen phlebotomy given weekly for several weeks bring hematocrit from 56 percent to a healthy 46 percent. We know physicians who prescribe phlebotomy once every six weeks because of an unusual response to testosterone replacement therapy. This is a simple procedure done in a hospital blood-draw facility that can reduce hematocrit, hemoglobin and blood iron immediately and easily in under one hour.

Prostate

A test for prostate specific antigen (PSA) should also be given to men over thirty-five years of age with a digital rectal exam. While several studies show that testosterone replacement is not associated with elevated PSA,[223][224] questions remain about the use of testosterone replacement for men who have prostate cancer, and there are questions about the use of supraphysiologic (ultra high) doses of testosterone and anabolic steroids related to prostate growth. As noted before, compelling data suggests that estrogen dominance may be a primary influence, so this should also be considered.[225] [226] Decreased progesterone has been cited as a possible factor, too.

Free Testosterone

While total testosterone is frequently the only measurement taken when hypogonadism is suspected, data strongly suggests that a free testosterone measurement is generally superior to total testosterone in evaluating testosterone function in both HIV(+) women and men.[227] For instance, free testosterone has been shown to be more correlative with optimal lean body mass than total testosterone in wasting HIV(+) men[228] and women.[212]

If the person has low free testosterone, he or she is a candidate for ongoing testosterone replacement therapy, whether or not they measure as having normal total testosterone. Sex-hormone binding globulin levels appear to increase throughout the course of HIV disease, and this progressively reduces the amount of free testosterone.[218]

It is important to do hormone testing in the morning on an empty stomach, as many things can affect free testosterone measurements, including diet. Elevated insulin caused by eating carbohydrates, for instance, can increase free testosterone levels by reducing plasma levels of sex-hormone binding globulin.[229]

Also consider that inadequate response to normal levels of free testosterone can be the result of marginal or frank nutritional deficiencies caused by inadequate nutrient intake or impaired nutrient absorption caused by gastrointestinal problems, like diarrhea. Optimizing nutrient intake by using dietary supplements and improving gastrointestinal health by eradicating any detected parasites will often elicit improved sensitivity to the body's own testosterone or supplemental testosterone. Optimal response means that lower doses of supplemental testosterone produce better results with less potential for side effects.

Other Hormones

We also suggest measuring DHEA, GH, IGF-1 and thyroid hormone for men and women, and estradiol, and progesterone for women. These tests can be done by blood tests or by using the easy, do-it-at-home mail order saliva hormone tests that are available without a prescription. Mail-order saliva tests for testosterone, DHEA, estradiol, cortisol and progesterone are offered by Great Smokies Laboratory. Call: 800-522-4762.

Bioelectrical Impedance Analysis (BIA)

BIA should be instituted when a person is diagnosed with HIV, and measurements should be taken every three to six months if the individual appears to be weight stable. Doctors should perform monthly BIA tests during the use of anabolic hormone cycles to ascertain the effectiveness of the steroids.

BIA can be valuable between steroid cycles, so that if the person begins to lose over 20 percent of the lean body mass that was gained during the steroid cycle, steps can be taken to obviate further loss.

According to the Merck Manual, normal free testosterone measurements for men generally range between 3.06 and 24 ng. per dL. Optimal free testosterone levels for men appear to be in the midrange or higher end of this scale. For women, the range is generally between .09 to 1.28 ng. per dL. Optimal free testosterone for women appears to be in the midrange of this scale.

Liver Function Tests

For HIV(+) people who have extremely compromised liver functions or Hepatitis C, and because many of the AIDS medications have liver toxic effects, physicians should carefully monitor liver function tests when oral steroids are used. These include standard multi-function tests such as SGOT, SGPT, and LDH, and the discreet liver tests – GGT, bilirubin, and the liver isoenzyme of LDH. One recent study asserts that GGT may be a more accurate indicator of steroid-induced liver problems than SGOT or SGPT.[230]

TYPES OF TESTOSTERONE REPLACEMENT

Males and females who are hypogonadal should be given continuous testosterone replacement therapy in one of three ways:

1. Prescription testosterone injections
2. Prescription transdermal testosterone cream or gel
3. Prescription testosterone patch.

Testosterone Injections

Injections are the most common type of replacement used by men, and are given at a weekly dose of about 100 to 200 mg. per week if testosterone is supplemented in its most common long-acting injectable forms, testosterone enanthate or testosterone cypionate. For women the dose range is from 2.5 to 20 mg. per week.

Injections have the advantage of once-per-week administration. Additionally, higher doses can be given to those men who appear to require higher blood levels, a common problem in highly progressed HIV(+) men. However, injections produce an unnaturally high blood testosterone level during the

first few days after injection. Then the blood level drops off each day and falls to baseline in about ten days. (See the chart below.) This doesn't effectively deliver normal blood levels of testosterone or mimic the natural daily pattern of testosterone release as well as gels, patches or creams can.

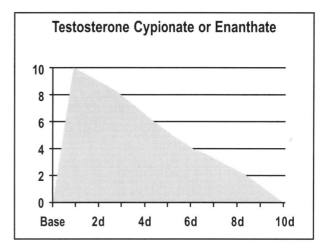

Source: Schulte-Beerbuhl, 1980[13]

Additionally, if we consider testosterone's effect as a stimulant of red blood cell production, injections produce unusually strong stimulation during the first day and for a few days thereafter. This appears to increase the potential for elevated hemoglobin (too many red blood cells), and hematocrit. Creams, gels and patches appear to have less potential to produce this side effect.

Anecdotally, we hear that injections promote elevations in blood pressure more than creams, gel, and patches. It also appears that the effect on brain chemistry and the nervous system that might promote aggressive behavior can be stronger with injections.

However, some HIV(+) men do appear to need the higher level of overall metabolic stimulation that injectable testosterone provides; there is no one-size-fits-all approach that works for everyone.

We also find that a very small subset of HIV(+) men appear to need brief rest periods of four to eight weeks with no testosterone injections because they become less sensitive to the effects of injectable testosterone after six to twelve months. This is something that a physician has to determine on a case-by-case basis by listening to the person's subjective feelings about their sexual function, energy, and overall feeling of well being. If they report that they are no longer experiencing the benefits of testosterone therapy, and raising the dose has been tried to no avail, then they may be well served by taking a short four- to eight-week break. Taking a break will usually help to return the person's sensitivity to the effects of testosterone injections.

However, we caution that people who really need to be on continuous replacement therapy can suffer a great loss of quality of life if they are taken off of testosterone, so the doctor should be sensitive to each person's evaluation of how they are feeling. If, a few weeks after the person breaks from replacement testosterone he or she is obviously tired, depressed, losing lean body mass, or feeling run down, it is probably time to begin administration of testosterone replacement therapy again. We see people for whom four weeks is enough break time, and others who seem to do well with eight weeks.

Testosterone Creams and Gels

We recommend considering the use of the testosterone creams and gels rather than injections for testosterone replacement therapy for both women and men. (Women generally prefer creams and men gels.) They appear to be considerably less idiosyncratic than injections because they produce more natural levels of testosterone without the high peak blood levels injections can cause.

Women's International Pharmacy recommends that creams or gels be applied two times per day: first thing in the morning, with a second dose applied twelve hours later. After a few weeks of twice daily application, a relatively-steady-state blood testosterone level is generally attained, according to pharmacist Kathy Lammers. Some doctors prescribe once-a-day application of creams or gels and feel that

this delivers a more natural effect. This application also occurs first thing in the morning to mimic the body's normal early morning rise in testosterone. Application to areas of the skin that have a layer of fat under them will slow the release of the testosterone so that blood levels are maintained longer. It is also recommended that the sites of application around the body are rotated so that optimal absorption is maintained. The best application areas include the stomach, the neck, the inner thighs, and the breasts. Be aware that some people complain about dark hair growth where the cream or gel is applied, especially if one site is used over and over again without rotation.

We also recommend creams or gels over patches because the amount of testosterone they contain per dose can be much higher than the 4, 5, and 6 mg. patches; as much as 90 mg. per gram. Additionally, patches cost about four times as much, with alcohol-based gels costing as little as $17 per month.

There are varying qualities of creams and gels made by compounding pharmacies around the United States, and some of the poorer quality products are gunky and flake off after they dry, so buy from a reputable pharmacy. The best gels are clear and basically disappear shortly after application. Most men prefer alcohol-based gels, which absorb through the skin better than water-based gels. Creams should not be greasy and should resemble good moisturizing creams.

Some good compounding pharmacies include: Women's International Pharmacy (800-279-5708), College Pharmacy (800-575-7776), Kronos Pharmacy (800-723-7455) and Applied Pharmacy Services (formerly GulfSouth) (877-729-1015), but there are many others around the United States and the world. Compounding pharmacies do not typically take insurance, so you have to request reimbursement from your insurance company.

Androgel, a very high quality prepackaged prescription testosterone gel made by UNIMED

Pharmaceuticals is available at pharmacies around the United States. Androgel is clean, clear, non-sticky, and odorless. It is available in 25-mg. or 50-mg. gel packs. It is about five times as expensive compared to compounded gels, so compounded products are preferred unless you have third party coverage that covers Androgel.

New in 2003, Testim, a testosterone gel made by Auxilium Pharmaceuticals, is available in 50 mg. tubes that have a resealable cap. Testim is clear and non-sticky with a slight musk-like fragrance. Although Testim is more expensive than compounded gels, it is about 10 percent less than Androgel at pharmacies around the United States.

Testosterone Patches – Men

Use of a testosterone patch like Alza's Testoderm or Smith/Kline Beecham's Androderm, or Alza's Testoderm TTS patches may be considered for men who need basic testosterone replacement therapy. Like gels, patches can be used to provide a base amount of testosterone when an anabolic steroid is used for weight gain.

Long-term use of Alza's older scrotal patch, Testoderm, might increase hair loss or prostate problems for some men, as one study stated that it causes increases in dihydrotestosterone (DHT) that are proportionately greater than the increase in testosterone because of enhanced 5-alpha reductase activity in scrotal skin.[231]

ALZA's newer patch, the TTS version of Testoderm, can be placed on other parts of the body, like the chest and back. While the Androderm patch can also be placed on other parts of the body, some people like the Testoderm TTS patch better because its glue is lighter and does not irritate skin the way the Androderm glue can. Still others think the Androderm is preferable because it sticks better and they report that they have no significant problem if "mineral oil or tea tree oil is used to clean the glue off."

We do not recommend patches used without an additional anabolic steroid for those who are wasting or need to gain muscle, as a study detailed at the NIH Wasting Syndrome Conference, May 20, 1997, at Bethesda, Maryland, showed that they are not effective for treatment of HIV-related wasting – the doses of the patches are too low. However, many people report improvements in libido, energy, and feeling of well being.

Replacement Doses May Not Reverse Wasting

Doses of steroids used for rapid, lean-body-mass increases are higher than a typical replacement dose of testosterone given for hypogonadism. Effective injectable testosterone replacement doses for HIV(+) men for maintenance are generally between 100 and 200 mg. per week. Rarely, we have seen men who are highly progressed who appear to require as much as 400 mg. per week to respond adequately, apparently because of hormonal insensitivity.

We agree with Dr. Jon Kaiser that sensitivity to many drugs including testosterone can be improved by optimal nutrient intake, gastrointestinal health, and optimal nutrient absorption, therefore making lower doses of replacement testosterone more effective. Using lower doses reduces the potential for side effects.

Recently a study by Coodley showed that there was no improvement in lean body mass in progressed men (less than 200 CD4 T cells) who had greater than 5 percent weight loss when they were given testosterone cypionate at 200 mg. every two weeks for three months.[232] This supports our concern that a 100 mg. per week standard testosterone replacement dose may be too low to effect a significant improvement in lean body mass for some progressed HIV(+) men. Consider that a testosterone replacement dose for hypogonadal HIV(–) men is generally about 100 mg. per week. Data in the published medical literature confirms that 100 mg. per week is not enough to create a significant anabolic (muscle-building) effect for HIV(−) men,[233] although it may be enough testosterone to give them feelings of normal quality of life.

Finding the Right Dose – Men

One problem an inexperienced doctor may encounter is finding the correct replacement dose to get the desired beneficial effects for HIV(+) patients. Within its therapeutic window, testosterone's possible side effects are not as serious as many other medications, but the doctor will get the best results with the least potential for significant side effects if he or she is careful in finding the optimal dosage for each individual patient.

We suggest starting with 100 mg. per week to see if the benefits of testosterone, including more energy and libido, and improved mood and appetite are experienced. If after four weeks there is not enough improvement, increase the weekly dose by 50 mg., and after four weeks on this regimen ask the person how they have responded. We also see a few men who do well with only 50 or 75 mg. per week, while 100 mg. causes problems. When the dose is too high the first noticeable side effects are usually oily skin and acne or irritability. If these occur, reduce the dose a little until the correct dose is found. The physician should also monitor changes in free testosterone, looking for correlations with their patient's reporting of his status.

The Normal Scale Does Not Seem to Apply to HIV(+) Men

We suggest that the physician focus on listening to the patient's reports of his status and free testosterone measurements because the standard normal range for total testosterone blood levels may be too low for HIV(+) men. In an article in the *Body Positive* newsletter (May 1994, page 22) regarding testosterone replacement for hypogonadal HIV(+) men, progressive researcher Judith Rabkin, Ph.D.,

of New York City, stated that in her study "those who experience significant improvements in sexual functioning tend to have higher serum testosterone levels, usually between 1,000 and 1,900 ng. per dL." (Remember, the normal scale for men is generally about 300 to 1,000 ng. per dL.) In private correspondence Dr. Rabkin stated that a few of the men in her study did respond at blood levels that were as low as 700 to 800 ng per dL. The important point is that "normal" is a relative term, especially as it relates to total testosterone measurements, and it generally does not apply well to HIV(+) men.

This was further supported in another study by Wagner and Rabkin that showed that HIV(+) men with clinical symptoms of testosterone deficiency who had testosterone levels that were not only in the normal range, but exceeded 500 ng./dl, responded to testosterone replacement therapy with significant improvements in libido (89 percent), in mood (67 percent), in energy (71 percent), and in appetite (67 percent).[234]

We suggest that if the patient is not responding appropriately to testosterone doses that deliver a free testosterone level in the low and even mid-range of the normal scale, the physician should consider working with doses that deliver measurements that register in the high end and sometimes above the upper limit of the normal scale. Optimum dosing can be very individual and it is best to be open to experimentation to find the dose that gets the desired effects of improvement in lean body mass, functional strength, energy, mood, increased appetite, and sexual function.

Physicians might also consider that the normal scale may be an inadequate measurement for HIV(+) people in general, whether they are hypogonadal or not. Thus we suggest that the physician listen to the patient directly rather than relying solely on the standard testing mechanisms and scales when making a determination of whether to prescribe testosterone replacement therapy and what supplemental hormone dosage is optimal. For women, the physician should exert great care in finding the optimal dose without overdosing, as women are significantly more prone to side effects than men. (See the section for women that follows.)

Testosterone Replacement Combined with an Anabolic Steroid

There are also individuals who function better, with less depression and more energy, when they use testosterone replacement therapy combined with an anabolic steroid. For them, injectable testosterone by itself produces less than optimal quality of life. For this use the anabolic steroid can be considered to be a metabolic stimulant with indirect antidepressive potential, in some respects similar to the use of compounds like classic antidepressive medications such as tricyclics, mono-amine oxidase inhibitors, and SSRI's (selective serotonin re-uptake inhibitors). A typical combination that produces this benefit is nandrolone decanoate added to testosterone, with the person complaining that testosterone alone makes them feel poorly, but when nandrolone is added they feel good. Nandrolone's effect on elevating dopamine is documented in the medical literature,[121-123] so it appears that this may be a valid treatment for patients who suffer from depression. We have seen this many times over several years, and suggest that the physician be sensitive to the patient's needs and consider this use.

STEROID CYCLING FOR MUSCLE GROWTH

Rationale Behind Cycling Anabolic Steroids

This section details the cycling approach, which is used for rapid weight gain. Cycling anabolic steroids is the backbone of the most effective program for gaining lean muscle tissue quickly for all

HIV(+) people who need to, but this is not in lieu of appropriate testosterone replacement. Even people who have normal healthy testosterone function should be given a replacement amount of testosterone as a hormone foundation when cycling nandrolone decanoate (Deca Durabolin), oxandrolone (Oxandrin), or stanozolol (Winstrol). The use of any effective steroids alone will cause a significant decrease in natural testosterone production (hypogonadism) and with it a decrease in the beneficial androgenic characteristics of testosterone that are required for optimal quality of life. This can result in decreased libido, energy, and appetite. Therefore, replacement testosterone should be given in conjunction with the use of any of these steroids. Oxymetholone (Anadrol), also, is best used with low dose testosterone, but it should generally be used with some caution when used with testosterone, as combining these two steroids increases the potential for side effects, like gynecomastia and hair loss. Testosterone at 50 to 100 mg. per week will generally provide appropriate replacement when Anadrol is used.

During the cycle individuals should do their best to eat high protein meals, get good rest, and exercise consistently to increase their lean body mass as quickly as possible to what is ascertained to be a healthy level. The total dose of testosterone and the anabolic steroid that is combined with it should be high enough to create an anabolic environment in the muscle tissue so that it responds optimally to the stimulation caused by exercise. The anabolic steroids are used to add anabolic potential to testosterone, without increasing the potential for the androgenic and estrogenic side effects that testosterone might cause if it was used by itself at higher than replacement doses.

12-Week Steroid Cycles

While some bodybuilding books detail complex anabolic steroid cycle patterns, most of the time the simplest cycles are the best. Effective cycles can employ constant low, medium, or high doses of one anabolic steroid or a combination of steroids, or the ramp pattern that is detailed below.

In the first example of steroid cycles, all of the recommended available steroids are added to a replacement dose of testosterone.

1. Nandrolone at 100 to 200 mg. per week added to 100 to 200 mg. of testosterone per week for twelve weeks.
2. Stanozolol at 4 mg. to 8 mg. three times per day added to 100 to 200 mg. of testosterone per week for twelve weeks.
3. Oxandrolone at 5 mg. to 10 mg. four times per day added to 100 to 200 mg. of testosterone per week for twelve weeks.
4. Oxymetholone at 12.5 mg. to 50 mg. two times per day for twelve weeks added to 50 to 100 mg. of testosterone per week for twelve weeks.

While anabolic steroid cycles are usually added to replacement doses of testosterone enanthate or testosterone cypionate injections, testosterone can also be administered as a transdermal cream, gel, or patch. Examples:

1. Oxandrolone at 5 mg. to 10 mg. four times per day added to 50 to 75 mg. of testosterone gel twice per day, 7.5 grams of Androgel per day or 5.0 grams of Testim per day;
2. Stanozolol at 4 mg. to 8 mg. three times per day added to 50 to 75 mg. of testosterone gel twice per day, 7.5 grams of Androgel per day or 5.0 grams of Testim per day;
3. Oxymetholone at 12.5 mg. to 50 mg. two times per day for twelve weeks added to 50 to 75 mg. of testosterone gel twice per day, 7.5 grams of Androgel per day or 5.0 grams of Testim per day.

Oral Steroids Increase Strength

Some doctors prescribe "stacking" cycles that combine an oral steroid with injectables, such as stanozolol or oxandrolone or oxymethone combined with nandrolone and testosterone.

Hypothetically, the effect of stacking an oral steroid with injectables may improve the total effect on muscle gain because 17-alpha alkylated oral steroids improve synthesis of muscle cell creatine (which improves overall muscle strength) significantly more than injectables.[235] There is also a possibility that increased creatine enhances muscle cell anabolic activity, but this is not known conclusively.

Ramp Cycles

Another type of cycle that resembles a ramp is utilized in the anabolic steroid cycles detailed below, including the high dose PoWeR cycle. The ramp approach, after an initial gradually escalating low-dose acclimation, plateaus at high doses during the middle weeks of the cycle, and then de-escalates the dosage gradually until cessation of the cycle to taper off the steroids. The purpose of this pattern is to ease up to the higher doses over a period of weeks gradually – some people feel wired or over-stimulated if they begin a cycle with high doses of anabolic steroids. During the middle high dose period be aware that you might have a tendency to be overly aggressive, or snappy. Catch yourself if you do and stay cool. The dose reduction in the final weeks allows you to ease off the steroids gradually because a few people experience a feeling of "crashing."

Oral steroids are most effective when taken in divided doses several times per day as they stay in the bloodstream for only a few hours after ingestion.

Moderate and Higher-Dose Ramp Cycles

As the table shows, the first suggested moderate-dose ramp cycle provides a base of 100 mg. of replacement testosterone plus 100 mg. of nandrolone decanoate for the first two weeks. The nandrolone dosage is increased from weeks three to nine to 200 mg. per week, for a basic moderate dosage, or 300 to 400 mg. for the person who still does not gain lean body mass adequately at 200 mg.

The higher dose cycle is similar to the moderate dose cycle, but uses even higher doses during the middle of the cycle.

If in early evaluation it has been determined that a hypogonadal patient requires 200 mg. of testosterone as a replacement dose, we suggest that testosterone be given as a 200 mg. dose rather than 100 mg. during the steroid cycle.

Higher Dose PoWeR Cycle

For high lean-body-mass gains when you have lost a significant amount of weight from an unexpected infection, we suggest implementing the PoWeR cycle, which is being administered by HIV doctors around the country. The PoWeR cycle is also useful for those who are severely underweight and want to develop and maintain a ready reserve of lean body mass. This can be extremely valuable if you experience an unexpected opportunistic infection with accompanying weight loss.

Joseph

Joseph was HIV(+) for six years when a bout with pneumonia caused him to drop from his normal weight of 185 pounds to 150 pounds (at 6'1" tall). To regain his weight he instituted a comprehensive high dose PoWeR cycle, and then over a period of two years used lower dose steroid cycles to build himself up to 235 pounds, which is an athletic level of lean body mass.

Joseph liked camping and the outdoors, and white water rafting was his one of his favorite releases. During one white-water rafting trip Joseph took a dip and ended up swallowing

water. Later that night he began to experience the beginning of a severe infection of cryptosporidium parvum, a water-borne pathogen, that lasted for over a month. During the crypto infection Joseph lost 50 lbs. before stabilizing at 185 lbs. If he had weighed 185 lbs. when he contracted the infection and lost 50 lbs., Dr. Donald Kotler's data suggests that Joseph might have had problems recovering or even surviving. Joseph thinks that anabolic steroids probably saved his life.

Joseph's story provides an argument for the institution of the PoWeR cycle to help an HIV(+) person build a reserve of quality lean body mass so that they have extra lean tissue to burn in case there is an unexpected illness.

It is important to note that wasting is generally a later stage condition that follows internal decline. Starting steroid therapy when early wasting is detected, which may occur before there is overt external wasting, may prevent or slow internal decline itself, and so the potential for the person to progress in HIV may be reduced considerably. There are also people who do not respond well enough to low and moderate dose cycles, and seem to require higher doses.

Nelson

Nelson Vergel, who had wasted to 140 lbs. in 1994, began his anabolic steroid therapy with a PoWeR cycle and put on thirty-five pounds of lean body mass in four months. All of his AIDS-related complex symptoms disappeared with the weight gain. After seventeen years of infection, Nelson currently weighs 196 pounds with only 7 percent body fat. Nelson stays on a maintenance program that consists of 100 mg. of testosterone cypionate and 200 mg. of nandrolone decanoate per week and has never had to use another PoWeR cycle. Most of the time his quality of life is excellent with tremendous productivity. His liver and kidney function are healthy and his PSA is low. His only problem is borderline high blood pressure, but he had this before using steroids.

PoWeR Ramp Cycle Table

The chart details what we suggest as a very high dose, highly effective anabolic steroid cycle that has the least potential for side effects. Options are given for the use of nandrolone, with a base amount of testosterone, at lower and higher doses. In the PoWeR cycle, if side effects like acne or irritability are experienced, it may help to reduce the highest dose of testosterone to only 100 or 200 mg., while increasing the nandrolone dosage to make up the total milligrams in the chart.

PoWeR Ramp Cycle Table

The chart details what we suggest as a very high dose, highly effective anabolic steroid cycle that has the least potential for side effects. Options are given for the use of nandrolone, with a base amount of testosterone, at lower and higher doses. In the PoWeR cycle, if side effects like acne and hair loss are experienced, it may help to reduce the highest dose of testosterone to only 100 or 200 mg., while increasing the nandrolone dosage to make up the total milligrams in the chart.

Men's Ramp Cycles

Cycle Week	1 — Moderate Nandrolone dosage (mg.) with base of testosterone	2 — Higher Dose Nandrolone dosage (mg.) with base of testosterone	The PoWer Cycle Testosterone enanthate or testosterone cypionate (T) combined with nandrolone decanoate (ND)
1	100 mg.	100 mg.	100 mg. T
2	100 mg.	100 mg.	200 mg. T + 100 mg. ND
3	200 mg.	200 mg.	300 mg. T + 200 mg. ND
4	200 mg.	200 mg.	300 mg. T + 200 mg. ND
5, 6, 7	200 mg.	300 mg. or 400 mg.	400 mg. T + 300 mg. ND
8	200 mg.	300 mg. or 400 mg.	300 mg. T + 300 mg. ND
9	200 mg.	200 mg.	200 mg. T + 200 mg. ND
10	200 mg.	200 mg.	100 mg. T + 200 mg. ND
11	100 mg.	100 mg.	100 mg. ND
12	100 mg.	100 mg.	100 mg. ND
13			
14			
21	Institute refraction guidelines on page 92 to return the body's natural testosterone production		

Moderate and higher dose cycles. These cycles address moderate weight loss. For some, #1 alone is effective enough to reach goal LBM. Others need #2 or #3. After the cycle, take a minimum sixteen-week break, monitoring every four weeks for LBM loss.

PoWeR cycle. For those who do not respond well enough to low or moderate dose cycles, or who have lost 10 percent of normal weight. Afterwards take a sixteen-week minimum break, monitoring every four weeks for LBM loss.

After the cycle if you lose 20 percent of the LBM gained during the cycle consider two options: either begin another cycle or add a low dose of a steroid like nandrolone (100 mg. per week), stanozolol (4 mg. three times per day), or oxandrolone (5 mg. four times per day) to ongoing testosterone replacement. For many people, testosterone replacement at 100 to 200 mg. per week will be enough to maintain weight.

Maintaining LBM Between Cycles

For people who have healthy testosterone production, we suggest a minimum sixteen-week period of total abstinence from any anabolic steroid, including testosterone, before instituting another cycle, unless you lose over 20 percent of the weight you gained during the steroid cycle. This gives the body time to resume natural testosterone production and reduces the potential for permanent inhibition of normal testosterone production.

It is essential that two critical components be maintained when the steroid cycle is ended to best maintain the lean body mass that was gained:

• First, the person should maintain consistent optimal protein intake, including eating meals with a high protein content and perhaps supplementing the diet with protein powder drinks. Remember that people who lift weights probably need a total of about 0.8 grams of protein per pound of body weight per day, according to data from Dr. Peter Lemon, of the University of Western Ontario.[236][237] We recommend 1 gram per pound to provide a margin for error. (People with liver or kidney problems should consult their doctor before increasing protein intake.)

• Second, a consistent weight-training program should be maintained. (See our suggestions in Chapter 25.)

Over the last few years, numerous hypogonadal people who clearly do not have adequate testosterone function have asked about cycling on and off all steroids, including testosterone. The majority of the time it is not appropriate for them to cycle off of testosterone, as they will experience a loss of lean body mass, energy, and overall quality of life. If anabolic steroids are used in addition to replacement testosterone in cycles by these people, maintenance testosterone replacement therapy should continue when the cycle of additional anabolic steroids ends.

While some people only have to use one PoWeR cycle to gain 20 or 35 pounds, they may need to institute another cycle at some time due to a bout with a catabolic illness that causes weight loss. Still some people only require replacement testosterone.

Cycling for People with Healthy Testosterone Function

There are also individuals who have healthy testosterone function yet have a medical reason to gain lean body mass. This might be because they are underweight to begin with, and increasing their lean body mass would contribute to their better overall physical and mental health, or because they have suffered from weight loss caused by a bout with an infection. These people do not need continuous testosterone replacement therapy after a steroid cycle ends.

Cycling is important for these people because cycling allows the body time to resume its normal testosterone production after the cycle is ended during the rest period. It also reduces long-term inhibition of the feedback loop that controls testosterone production in the body.

Dr. Shalender Bhasin of UCLA told us that it took no longer than sixteen weeks (four months) for healthy HIV(–) men to return to normal testosterone production after his 600 mg. per week ten-week testosterone enanthate study.[238] He also confirms that the return to normal took no more than six months for the healthy men in his male contraceptive study that employed 200 mg. of testosterone enanthate per week for one year. While long-term, very high dose steroid or testosterone abuse could elicit a more negative result and take even longer to return to normal, and may even cause a permanent inhibition of testosterone production, Dr. Bhasin's statement suggests that the body will resume its natural testosterone production after the use of the medically sound and reasonable steroid doses we recommend. Whether HIV(+) men have less potential for a full return of normal testosterone production is not known, however.

REFRACTION GUIDELINES – MEN

Helping the Body Quickly Return Testosterone Production to Normal

(For men who were not hypogonadal when they started.)

All steroids cause the body to turn down its own testosterone production shortly after you start using them, and testosterone production does not return to normal immediately after you stop using them. "Refraction" refers to the period of time after the use of steroids when the body continues to produce less testosterone than normal. Without intervention with our refraction guidelines it can take three to six months to have normal testosterone production again, assuming it was normal to start with. But with these guidelines we have seen testosterone productions return to full normal levels after as little as two weeks.

Testosterone and Immune Function

Returning the body's testosterone production to normal quickly is important for those men whose bodies can produce normal levels of testosterone. When testosterone is low there can be an imbalance in the normal testosterone-to-cortisol relationship that favors cortisol, an immunosuppressive, catabolic hormone, as the dominant hormone. Testosterone and cortisol, in some aspects, are counter-balancing hormones in their effects on the immune system and muscle tissue. Reduced testosterone can allow cortisol to depress immune function, and can break down muscle tissue. We know that cortisol depresses T-cell production and catabolizes muscle, while testosterone supports healthy T-cell metabolism and builds muscle.

We have seen bodybuilders coming off steroid cycles contract infections (especially upper respiratory infections), probably because cortisol, as an immunosuppressive hormone, weakens certain critical immune functions. This is one reason that it is important to quickly restore testosterone levels after cessation of a cycle.

Remember, this refraction protocol is for men whose bodies can produce normal levels of testosterone. It is not for men who are clinically hypogonadal before the use of steroids. If you are truly hypogonadal you should stay on testosterone replacement when you come off the cycle.

The Refraction Guidelines Cocktail

These three medications complement each other:

1. **HCG (human chorionic gonadotropin)**

    HCG mimics luteinizing hormone (LH), the natural hormone in your body that tells the testes to produce testosterone. If the testicles have atrophied (shrunken) during the steroid cycle, they will likely begin to enlarge and up-regulate their testosterone production significantly shortly after HCG therapy is instituted. HCG "jump-starts" the testes.

    While we have heard it stated that HCG addresses testicular function rather than brain center control of leutinizing hormone (LH), one study has shown that while HCG increased testosterone production, it also increased LH significantly.[239]

    We note that HCG may have therapeutic benefits for Kaposi's Sarcoma[240] and HCG's beta unit has anti-HIV activity in vitro.[241]

    Administration: HCG is a water-based injectable medication, rather than an oil-based medication like common injectable steroids, so small

29-gauge ultra-fine syringes can be used rather than the larger (more painful) 22-gauge needles required for steroid injections. Most men inject HCG into the top of the thigh while seated. Ask your doctor for instructions on how to inject. HCG dosing is either of two patterns: More men report that they prefer the perceived effect of 5,000 IU once per week for four weeks; another option is 2,000 IU every other day for fourteen injections. (One vial contains 10,000 IU.) Some men experience bloating, moodiness, acne, or hair loss when they use the 5,000 IU pattern, but they find that the 2,000 IU pattern causes no problems. (While a majority of men report that the 5,000 IU pattern feels as if it is more effective for stimulating testosterone production, some published data indicates that lower doses, such as 1,500 IU, are just as effective.)

Note: HCG can also be used by itself during the middle of an anabolic steroid cycle to reverse testicular atrophy (shrunken testicles). This method employs an injection of 5,000 IU of HCG followed one week later by another 5,000 IU during the approximate midpoint of the cycle, or any time that the testes appear to have shrunken.

2. Arimidex (anastrozole)

Arimidex, an antiestrogen, reduces estrogen production by inhibiting the activity of aromatase, the enzyme that converts testosterone to estrogen. Since the hypothalamus senses estrogen as one of the primary barometers it uses to determine how much testosterone to produce,[242] the decrease in estrogen induced by Arimidex signals the hypothalamus to increase leutinizing hormone releasing hormone. This causes increased production of leutinizing hormone, which in turn stimulates the leydig cells in the testes to produce testosterone.

Arimidex is a good partner compound to be used when HCG is used, because HCG can also increase estrogen and the potential for estrogen-related side effects substantially. Arimidex inhibits this effect.

Administration: Arimidex is taken at 1 mg. per day during the two-month refraction protocol. Caution: Arimidex should generally not be used at 1 mg. per day for longer than is necessary, as estrogen is required for healthy brain chemistry and cardiovascular health, so long-term inhibition can cause health problems. Long-term use to reduce estrogen in men is typically at a lower dose, such as 1/2 tablet every other day, as determined by testing.

3. Clomid (clomiphene citrate)

Clomid, another type of antiestrogen, can have a pronounced effect on return of important quality of life functions like libido, and feelings of well being.[243] Clomid increases luteinizing hormone and testosterone, but does not appear to down-regulate testicular leydig cell activity, because it blocks testicular estrogen receptors as an estrogen antagonist.[240]

We caution that some men may experience mood changes and feel more emotional when using Clomid. For them, HCG and Arimidex can be used for the full eight weeks without Clomid. This should still produce a full restoration of testicular function. Over time, monitoring many individuals, we have seen what appears to be less benefit from the use of Clomid than HCG, overall. Clomid can be quite expensive, so you may choose not to employ it.

Administration: 50 mg. of Clomid is taken two times per day starting on day 29, after HCG administration ceases.

If your health insurance does not cover clomiphene or HCG, a good low-price source for them in the United States is Applied Pharmacy

Services Call them at 877-729-1015 or go to: www.appliedpharmacyrx.com

Testing

At the end of twenty-eight days we suggest testing free and total testosterone levels to ascertain how well the person is responding to this protocol. We also suggest testing again at the end of this protocol in two months and again in three months.

Growth Hormone for Refraction

Low dose GH administration may increase the effectiveness of the refraction guidelines because GH has been shown to improve the response of ley-dig cells to leutinizing hormone.[244] This improves testosterone production. Our suggested dose for this use is 0.5 mg. (1.5 IU) per day before bedtime during the refraction protocol.

Note: HCG/Arimidex/Clomid therapy is not a perfect way to re-institute normal testosterone production quickly, but it can work very well.

GUIDELINES FOR WOMEN

Natural Hormone Replacement Therapy (HRT)

At the NIH Wasting Conference in Bethesda, Maryland, on May 20, 1997, Dr. Donald Kotler explained that gender is correlative with differences in changes in body composition in wasting. Women tend to lose fat sooner than men in the process of wasting, and also regain fat quickly after recovery from opportunistic infections, and this is logically a result of differences in hormone levels in men and women; since men have higher testosterone levels and lower estrogen levels than women, it is easier for men to maintain more lean muscle mass with lower body fat.

We suggest that a complete natural hormone replacement therapy (HRT) program monitored by a knowledgeable doctor should be considered for all women living with HIV, especially if lean tissue loss is detected by DEXA or BIA, if hormone analysis (saliva or blood) shows that hormone levels are inadequate, or if a woman experiences irregular menstrual cycles or lack of menstruation, a symptom of hormonal deficiency. While in the past, HRT addressed only estrogen, optimal HRT for women with HIV should take into consideration estradiol, progesterone, DHEA, testosterone, and thyroid, as each of these interdependent hormones can have a role in maintaining lean body mass and overall health. For example, decreasing DHEA levels are associated with decreasing free testosterone levels and decreasing lean body mass in late-stage HIV(+) women.[212] Replacement doses of DHEA will also provide a significant increase in testosterone in women (but not in men[245]) so that testosterone replacement is sometimes not necessary. See also the section on DHEA that follows.

Employing complete natural HRT becomes more compelling when we see that one study suggests that HRT as estrogen alone may increase the risk of death in HIV(+) women.[246] While this information has not been investigated in depth, physicians should consider that HIV disease progression may be increased by hormonal imbalance – too little of some hormones (testosterone, DHEA, and progesterone) relative to too much estrogen may create what amounts to a pro-inflammatory metabolism. It is known that, in women, a deficiency of testosterone, or an imbalance between testosterone and estrogen with relatively too much estrogen, may increase progression of other immune pathologies like the autoimmune disease lupus.[208] HIV likely has a similar potential.

After hormone testing is completed to ascertain replacement strategies, compounding pharmacies like Women's International Pharmacy (800-279-

5708) can create whatever natural transdermal HRT cream formula is required for each individual. Call them to get an information packet that you can share with your doctor. Transdermal creams deliver hormones by being absorbed through the skin (dermis). Transdermal creams are gentler and safer than tableted HRT drugs.

If lean tissue status cannot be maintained by complete hormone replacement therapy alone, we suggest that an aggressive anabolic steroid program, like the ones outlined below, be added.

New HRT Information (January 2003)

PremPro, the most commonly prescribed form of oral HRT in the United States was shown in a large government sponsored study to increase the risk of breast cancer 26 percent, heart disease 22 percent, heart attacks 29 percent, venous blood clots 100 percent and strokes 41 percent.[247] [248] [249] Perhaps part of the reason PremPro caused some of these problems is because PremPro is not composed of natural hormones. PremPro consists of two hormones: horse estrogens (Premarin) that include one form of estrogen that is not made in the human body; and medroxyprogesterone (Progest), a laboratory-created created analog to the natural hormone progesterone.

We suggest considering only natural HRT creams. Natural HRT has not been studied to see if it causes these problems, but an indepth analysis of the biochemistry involved suggests that natural HRT would have considerably less potential to cause some of the problems PremPro use is associated with. Please share this information with your doctors for their consideration.

Low-Dose Steroid Cycle for Women

After hormone replacement therapy is determined, the oral anabolic steroid oxandrolone can be used at 2.5 mg. to 5 mg. two times per day for twelve

weeks or until the target body weight is achieved. A small subset of women could experience some virilizing (oily skin, acne, facial hair growth, deeper voice, and itching clitoris followed by clitoral growth) from this normally very safe and gentle steroid. If this happens, reduce the dosage immediately or stop.

Stanozolol in doses of 2 mg. to 4 mg. two times per day can also be used, but it presents somewhat more potential for virilizing effects.

Higher-Dose Steroid Cycles for Women

Higher-dose cycles should be considered for women who need quick increases in lean body mass. Steroid options include oxandrolone, stanozolol, nandrolone and oxymetholone. We suggest oxandrolone at 20 mg. per day for twelve weeks. Or stanozolol can be used at an equal or lower dose (12 mg. per day) with somewhat more potential for virilizing. Some HIV(+) women have used oxymetholone at as much as 25 mg. per day. We suggest caution when oxymetholone is used by women, although it appears to be safer than we thought initially. If you have a very urgent need to gain lean body mass, nandrolone decanoate can be added at 25 to 50 mg. per week. Nandrolone does present significantly more potential for virilizing, so monitoring for androgenic side effects is essential if it is used.

=====

GUIDELINES FOR MEN AND WOMEN
Serostim Human Growth Hormons (GH)

In the 1980s human growth hormone was the first anabolic drug to be embraced by AIDS activists to address wasting, the number two cause of death in AIDS. At that time, media hype and a hysterical anti-drug political climate created an exaggerated image of anabolic steroids as dangerous immuno-suppressive drugs that had no legitimate medical uses. For this reason the medical community and some leading AIDS activists rejected any consideration of the use of anabolic steroids and instead attached their hope to GH, which we assert was an error that delayed the understanding and acceptance of the beneficial use of anabolic steroids for HIV. It is interesting to note that the FDA panel that was to decide whether to approve GH deadlocked because of a lack of convincing data of its effectiveness and only approved it after AIDS activists showed their extreme support. Another interesting point is that it appears that the biotech company, Genentec, decided not to seek approval for their GH product because they did not feel that it would be effective for this use. With all this considered, GH has apparently produced life-saving effects for some HIV(+) people who were near death and we believe that it does have a place in treatment of body composition problems in HIV therapy. An analysis of many years of published data strongly suggests that GH does not have a direct effect on muscle tissue growth.[250] [251] [252] [253] [254] However, it may be that GH improves the health of some organ tissues that affect muscle growth. And so, some people with severe wasting may experience a small amount of muscle growth, re-hydration and improved organ function with GH therapy. However, GH is marketed inappropriately as a muscle builder, where anabolic steroids are far more effective. As will be discussed later, GH's primary value is its effect on fat cell metabolism.

Comparison of Anabolic Steroids and Growth Hormone

What the table on page 97 graphically illustrates is the tremendous disparity between the different anabolic compounds for lean body mass gained versus price. While nandrolone decanoate yielded as much as 11.88 pounds of lean body mass over fifteen weeks at a cost of approximately $150 per month or less, a 6 mg. (18 IU) daily dose of Serostim GH, which cost about forty times more than nandrolone, yielded only a little over half as much lean body mass after twelve weeks. Low doses of other steroids produced equal or better results than Serostim, for much less cost. Even Oxandrin, which is overpriced at $900 per month for 20 mg. per day, outperformed Serostim. Additionally, it is likely that the LBM gained from the steroids consisted of considerably more muscle tissue than was gained with Serostim. A majority of weight gain from Serostim has been shown to be water. (See the section below titled, "Growth Hormone Gains: Little Muscle, Lots of Water.")

Some studies report only total weight (Wt), not lean body mass (LBM) or body cell mass (BCM). Given this, we present the limited available data. Note: BCM is the metabolically active tissue that includes muscle and organs like the heart, liver, and kidneys. LBM includes BCM, connective tissue, water and bone. Total weight includes LBM and fat.

Choices: Serostim, Oxandrin, Anadrol, or Winstrol

For cost versus weight gain, testosterone and nandrolone are the best anabolic agents without a doubt. Just as it is clear that GH is out of the running in a contest for effect on lean body mass gains versus cost, Oxandrin used alone doesn't score much better. Although the men in the Poles study did gain 6.9 pounds of body cell mass on 20 mg. of Oxandrin per day over eight weeks, a chart review of wasting HIV(+) males by Dr. Patricia Salvato showed a weight gain of under two pounds with 20 mg. per day over twelve weeks.[255] Our real-world experience is that many male patients need 30 to 50 mg. per day of Oxandrin to gain significant LBM if it is used alone. A 30 to 50 mg. daily dose of Oxandrin costs $1.50 per milligram or $1,350 to $2,250 per month in the U.S. Oxandrolone (or any steroid) will produce much

Comparison of U.S. Anabolic Agents – Cost Versus Weight Gain

Anabolic Agent	Author Year	Study Length in Weeks	Number of Subjects	Exercise	Dose (mg.)	Average Weight Gain in Pounds	Cost per Month
Nandrolone	Gold 1996	16	17	Yes	100 mg. every 2 weeks	6.6 – Wt	$16
Nandrolone	Bucher 1996	12	73	No	100 mg./week	5 – BCM	$32
Testosterone Enanthate	Bhasin 1996	10	43	Yes	600 mg./week	13.42 – LBM	$29
Nandrolone & Testosterone	Salvato 1997	12	20	No	Escalating – De-escalating 100-700 mg./wk	13 – Wt	$70 Average
Nandrolone	Strawford 1997 2nd phase, 12 wks	1st phase, 3 wks 2nd phase 12 wks	18	No	1st – 195 mg. per wk (3 wks), then 2nd – 200 mg. every 2 wks	1st – 5.28 2nd – 6.6 Total 11.88 LBM	$38 Average
Winstrol	Berger 1993	10	1	No	6 mg./day	10 – Wt	$72
Winstrol	Berger 1993	4	1	No	6 mg./day	3.5 – Wt	$72
Oxandrin	Poles 1997	8	21	No	20 mg./day	6.9 – BCM	$900
Anadrol	Hengge 1996	30	30	No	150 mg./day	18 – Wt	$1080
Serostim GH	Schambelan 1996	12	178	No	6 mg./day	6.6 – LBM	$6000

better results if combined with testosterone. That is why a very tightly controlled eight-week study by Strawford that included comprehensive weight training showed that 10 mg. of oxandrolone twice per day combined with 100 mg. of testosterone per week increased lean body mass by 15.18 pounds compared to 8.36 pounds for testosterone alone with weight training. We note that 100 mg. of testosterone alone producing 8.36 pounds of weight gain is exceptional – this has never been seen before in any study of testosterone like this. We know these researchers to be among the very best at creating tightly controlled studies, and the results of this study were exceptional most probably because the authors did an extraordinary job creating the study and executing it. So, comparison of the results of this study to others is difficult. Our real-world experience and reports from HIV(+) men makes us assert that oxandrolone is probably the least potent of the available anabolic steroids, and this opinion is supported by an overview of the results of all the other studies of oxandrolone in HIV.

The only HIV study of the most potent oral anabolic steroid, Anadrol, does not give good representation of its cost versus benefit. The 1996 Hengge study of thirty patients over thirty weeks showed that 150 mg. per day of Anadrol produced an average of 18 pounds of weight gain. It should also be noted that the subjects in the Hengge study continued to gain weight, even during periods of illness. Anadrol, at this dose, would cost $1,080 per month in the U.S. However, these numbers are somewhat confusing. At 24 cents per milligram Anadrol is the most cost-effective oral anabolic steroid, and a 150 mg. daily dose is not necessary for the majority of HIV(+) males. It is possible that at 25 mg./day ($180 per month) or 50 mg./day ($360 per month) Anadrol can increase lean body mass equal to or better than equal doses of Oxandrin, and easily exceed any anabolic effect of GH, but at a much lower cost than either of these compounds. Based

on credible anecdotes, it is likely that even 10 to 20 mg. of Anadrol per day will increase lean body mass 5 to 10 pounds over twelve weeks. If weight training were included, the lean body mass gain could be even greater.

While Anadrol has a reputation for being a powerful steroid with a significant potential for side effects and liver toxicity, its historic use has been in ultra-high daily doses of 100 mg. or more for long periods of time as treatment for anemia. Doctors report liver toxicity when Anadrol is used in HIV at doses of 100 mg. per day and especially 150 mg. per day. It is likely that any oral anabolic steroid used long term at ultra high doses will produce side effects and liver toxicity that will not be seen with short term or low dose administration. Used at a low dose of 25 mg. per day in twelve-week cycles, the potential for side effects is reduced considerably, while low doses will still promote significant weight gain. The 50 mg. Anadrol tablets are scored in half, so consider splitting the tablet into doses of one-quarter-tablet and take one-quarter-tablet two or three times per day if you choose to try a low dose. (Remember, for best effect, oral steroids should be taken in divided doses several times per day, as blood levels decline after only a few hours.) It is likely that even one-half tablet per day would produce some muscle gain.

The other oral steroid, Winstrol, should also be considered. Winstrol produces good increases in lean body mass with little potential for side effects at a relatively low cost of 40 cents per milligram.[256] Berger's study of 6 mg. of Winstrol per day showed good weight gain,[256] which might suggest that it may produce more anabolic activity than a comparable dose of Oxandrin, as a similar Berger HIV study did not show any weight gain with 5 mg. of Oxandrin per day.[257] Winstrol also exerts its greatest effect when combined with testosterone. It also has not exhibited significant liver toxicity in the few HIV(+) men we know who have used it at standard low doses. Unfortunately,

Winthrop, the manufacturer of Winstrol in the U.S., has taken no interest in marketing it to the HIV community or supporting studies. For this reason, we rarely hear of doctors prescribing it.

The Politics of Serostim Growth Hormone

While appropriately prescribed human growth hormone can be another valuable tool in HIV therapy for the war against wasting and especially lipodystrophy as fat gain, we have considerable philosophical problems with the financial politics related to GH, and are quite critical of its exorbitant price and the deceptive way that it is marketed to the HIV community. Serostim, the GH product that has been approved for AIDS wasting therapy, costs over $6,000 per month for a full 6 mg. daily dose. This is about thirty-five times as expensive as the PoWeR cycle that employs high doses of testosterone and nandrolone. But is GH as effective for lean body mass gains for HIV(+) people? The study-comparison table above indicates that it is not. We also note that while compassionate use patient access programs from BTG and UNIMED are easy to work with, Serono's compassionate use program for people who do not have insurance is not.

Serostim Growth Hormone Has No Preservative

Even if the high cost of Serostim for the relatively small increase in lean body mass was not an issue, another problem with Serostim *is* important. Serono omits including a bacteriostatic agent in the sterile water that Serostim is reconstituted with, so it must be used within twenty-four hours after mixing or thrown away because bacteria might grow in the solution. This makes Serostim much more profitable for Serono, while it effectively takes away your option of reducing common side effects by rationing out part of the vial every day to get a lower side-effect-free daily dose.

If Serono did include a preservative like benzyl alcohol or metacresol in the mixing water, then you could use whatever dose was found to be appropriate, and store the unused GH in the refrigerator for up to two weeks. Currently, HIV(+) individuals who cannot tolerate the severe side effects that the full 4, 5, or 6 mg. doses can cause may end up throwing away any GH that they cannot use. More drug is wasted and thus more drug is sold.

Serono clearly knows about this issue, as their GH product called Saizen, which is sold in Mexico and Italy and prescribed to children in the U.S., does have benzyl alcohol in its mixing water. We had a discussion about this with Serono's director of research in 1997 and were told that it was too difficult to access an effective preservative. To this day Serono representatives have been evasive about the lack of a preservative.

Extending Serostim's Lifespan

One way to correct Serostim's lack of a preservative is to get your doctor to give you a prescription for bacteriostatic water that includes benzyl alcohol (made by Abbott Labs and other companies). An insider at Serono admitted that mixing Serostim with bacteriostatic water would allow it to be used for up to two weeks after mixing. After all, Serostim is essentially the same product as the other GH called Saizen, except that Saizen comes with bacteriostatic water that contains benzyl alcohol. Using bacteriostatic water allows you to find your own side-effect-free individual daily dose without waste.

Reducing Side Effects

If GH is given as a replacement hormone to HIV(–) people who are GH deficient or are experiencing an age-related decrease in GH production, the typical daily dose is around .5 mg. (1.5 IU) per day. Bodybuilders know about safe, side-effect-free doses and typically limit their use of GH to under 1.4 mg. (about 4 IU) per day.

Serostim is currently packaged in doses of 4, 5, or 6 mg. vials, and a study of the medical literature show that these doses are overdoses for many people. Doses that are this high can cause significant side effects including arthralgia (joint pains), carpal tunnel syndrome, edema (water retention), elevated blood sugar, elevated pancreatic enzymes, gynecomastia, body hair growth, and high blood pressure.

Serono's dosing recommendations are lacking in that they instruct patients to use one full vial per day. If this causes side effects the doctor often tells the person to use the full vial every other day, or use only part of the vial every other day, and throw the rest away. These instructions are inadequate. Doctors who work with GH for anti-aging purposes tell us that GH has very little potential for side effects if it is administered in smaller doses more often, with the best effect being seen with twice-a-day administration. Without the peak blood levels that high doses every other day create, there will be fewer side effects. In general, with any drug, smaller doses given more often work better with fewer side effects than large doses given less often. Our recommendation for best effect is to administer GH first thing in the morning and once before bed. If this is too much trouble, administer it before bedtime.

GH and Joint Inflammation

Significant research shows that high dose GH may cause joint pains because it can promote excess super oxide secretion by neutrophils, which causes inflammation.[258] [259] This effect has a known association with inflammatory joint problems, such as rheumatoid arthritis,[260] so high dose GH appears to be inducing a state like rheumatoid arthritis.

Richard's Response to GH

We have seen a few HIV(+) individuals who have a seemingly tremendous anabolic response to the use of high dose GH, and much more so than they do to anabolic steroids. This can be deceptive.

For instance, one of our close friends, Richard, who was fifty-five years old and had been extremely progressed in AIDS (several times near death), was an example of a person who had a significantly poor response to the effects of anabolic steroids, as steroids have not helped him gain as much lean body mass as some people do. In an attempt to help him gain weight, his doctor put him on Serostim GH, and two weeks after he had started Serostim we were surprised to find that he had gained eighteen pounds. (We even thought that we might have to re-assess our somewhat critical position on GH.)

However, a few days into his third week he began to be overwhelmed by the problems he was having with side effects. It seems that because of his hopes that GH would be the magic bullet that it is advertised as, he had down-played the fact that he had been experiencing extreme swelling and pain in his hands and other joints, numbness in his hands and arms when he slept, difficulty breathing when he climbed stairs, and he was unable to sleep on his back because he felt like he was suffocating.

On examination, his doctor found that most of the weight he had gained was water, and determined that he was suffering from severe pulmonary edema (water in the lung tissues), so she immediately admitted him to the hospital. After several critical medical procedures while he was in the hospital - he was almost given open-heart surgery - he recovered to live another day. His doctor said that it is unlikely that she would prescribe Serostim again. We assert that this kind of situation can result from the use of the currently recommended 4, 5, and 6 mg. doses that for most people are overdoses of GH, and the fact that there is no preservative in Serostim's formulation, which deters people from lowering their dose to reduce the side effects.

Growth Hormone Gains: Little Muscle, Lots of Water

When all things are considered, it appears that Serono recommends what amounts to an overdose of GH because an ultra-high overdose is necessary to come close to producing lean body mass (LBM) gains that seem to be almost equal to the anabolic effects of low doses of anabolic steroids. Using GH to grow muscle is an incorrect use; the increase in LBM may very well consist primarily of water, with some connective tissue, a little organ tissue, and only a little, if any, muscle tissue.

Indeed, one carefully designed study of high-dose GH with HIV(–) young men used sophisticated techniques to closely examine the composition of the lean tissue gained and concluded that it consisted of lean tissue other than muscle.[250] This could mean water, connective tissue, and organ tissue. At least five other studies with other populations have also shown an increase in LBM, but a lack of muscle growth.[251 252 261 262 263] It should be noted that Dr. Kathleen Mulligan stated that GH-induced lean body mass gains for HIV patients were "comparable" to the healthy HIV(–) controls in her study,[264] so comparisons with studies of HIV(–) subjects may very well be valid.

Indeed, the first HIV study that looked at Serostim using magnetic resonance imaging (MRI), a sophisticated technology that actually looks at what is happening to the body's tissues, indicated that growth hormone may have little or no affect on muscle. At the Third International Conference on Nutrition and HIV Infection at Cannes, France, in April, 1999, Dr. Donald Kotler reported the results of an interim analysis of a six-month open-label trial of Serostim growth hormone that showed that 6 mg. per day did not promote a significant change in muscle tissue during the first twelve weeks in the eight subjects for whom repeat MRI data was available. Final study results showed what appeared to be an increase. However, this study's lack of a placebo control makes its data inconclusive. It appears that if Serostim does actually have an effect on increasing muscle tissue through direct or indirect means, it does so erratically and only for a very few HIV(+) people, not for the majority.

GH and Gynecomastia

Gynecomastia is the growth of breast tissue in men. It is sometimes seen in males who use high doses of anabolic steroids that aromatize into estro-gen, as estrogen stimulates breast tissue growth. Gynecomastia appears to be a very rare phenomenon in HIV(+) men, at least partially because impaired insulin-like growth factor-1 (IGF-1) production and GH deficiency are common in HIV,[265 266] and IGF-1 is a necessary cofactor with estrogen for breast tissue growth in gynecomastia.[267 268] GH stimulates production of IGF-1 by the liver, and our observation is that HIV(+) males who use growth hormone appear to have a much higher incidence of gynecomastia than those who don't. Indeed, older studies with young HIV(–) boys and senior men who receive growth hormone therapy have documented incidence of gynecomastia.[269 270] GH can also stimulate breast tissue growth by binding to prolactin receptors.[271]

Measurements: Finding the Right GH Dosage

Analysis of the available data causes us to assert that GH should be considered for replacement purposes based on blood tests, rather than as a muscle growth stimulant, and prescribed accordingly. However, no studies have been done to ascertain what blood levels are appropriate for HIV(+) males and females. Until this is done, our suggestion is that the physician consider testing IGF-1, which is a more consistent measurement than plasma GH, and try to arrive at an IGF-1 measurement of approximately 350 ng./mL, which is the target reading for optimal GH replacement for anti-aging purposes. Because hormonal resistance is common in HIV, it is possible that some HIV(+) people will require higher blood levels to experience the potential improvements in fat metabolism and quality of life. To date we have seen doses of between 0.5 mg. and 3 mg. per day produce optimal effects for HIV(+) men, so we suggest starting at 0.5 mg. per day, and retesting to work toward determining an appropriate dose. Also, doctors are advised to listen to your patients' subjective reports of their status to determine what is optimal, and be willing to experiment until you find what is appropriate.

Growth Hormone's Benefits

While the available data suggests that GH is not anabolic to muscle tissue like anabolic steroids, and it is clear that GH's price and Serono's lack of a preservative do not serve the HIV(+) population, GH does have unique benefits. If GH has more effect on increasing the growth of lean tissue other than muscle, as the studies suggest, does it promote the regeneration of organ tissue like the thymus, kidneys, and liver? This is an area that needs to be researched. Wasting in HIV is not limited to muscle tissue, and regeneration of critical organs in the body may be an important reason for GH replacement therapy in HIV. As was said, it may be that the rare anecdotal reports of a small amount of increased muscle growth in severely wasted HIV(+) individuals are the result of improved function of organs that indirectly affect muscle growth.

And, while anabolic steroids can reduce the net ratio of fat to muscle that is gained[272] and can have some effect on increasing the loss of fat, GH's most important effect may be its role in fat cell metabolism;[273] it increases lipid oxidation (fat burning),[274] which gives it a role in possible therapies to reduce some of the symptoms of the bodyfat redistribution, called "lipodystrophy." Dr. Gabe Torres documented that GH can reduce bodyfat gained in the abdominal area and this is an area that we feel should be investigated thoroughly.

However, we caution that GH may increase the loss of subcutaneous fat on the arms, legs, and face, which is the part of lipodystrophy syndrome called "lipoatrophy."

The role of human growth hormone (GH) is also interesting when we consider that a phenomenon of early AIDS wasting is the loss of muscle, while fat is gained, described as *de novo lipogenesis* by Dr. Marc Hellerstein.[275] This kind of catabolism of muscle and anabolism of fat is somewhat unique to AIDS, and it may be in part caused by a resistance to GH[276] and reduced production of IGF-1.[277] So, GH appears to have a unique role in a problem that is somewhat specific to AIDS.

We also have anecdotal reports that growth hormone use sometimes stops chronic diarrhea. GH is known to increase tissue regeneration in the intestine[278] and improve intestinal water and ion absorption,[279] so this is possible.

GH Combined with Anabolic Steroids

GH may have valuable adjunctive benefits when used to address GH deficiency when it is combined with testosterone replacement therapy. Appropriately-dosed GH replacement may also enhance the effectiveness of any of the PoWeR anabolic steroid cycles, just as nutritional supplementation that addresses nutrient deficiencies does. We invite the research community to study combination therapy that employs GH replacement and anabolic steroids.

Hyperplasia

When GH is added to a regimen of anabolic steroids and weight training it seems that what muscle is gained is more permanent than when anabolic steroids are used alone. This may be because GH's effect of increasing IGF-1 can increase the number of nuclei in muscle cells by causing satellite cells to fuse to adjacent muscle cells or differentiate into muscle cells.[280] This might result in hyperplasia, an increase in the number of muscle cells, and hypertrophy, an increase in cell size. Observation of bodybuilders suggests that this effect may be potentiated by proper exercise stimulus and optimal levels of androgens. (Note: GH used by itself does not appear to produce lasting lean tissue gains after administration is stopped.[281] This would be true if most of the weight that was gained was water.)

Doctor to Doctor

Physicians might be interested in hearing the experience of another physician who is familiar with the use of anabolic steroids as detailed in this chapter. For this, you might call any of several clinicians who are familiar with our approach. These include: in Houston, Patricia Salvato, M.D. (713-960-7900) and Shannon Schrader, M.D. (713-520-5537); in Los Angeles, Tony Mills, M.D. (310-550-1010). These doctors report that many patients using the PoWeR cycle have gained twenty to forty pounds with increased energy and greatly improved quality of life in a matter of two to four months without significant side effects.

These physicians also report some improvements in some of the symptoms of lipodystrophy using specific elements of our program, including reduced visceral fat and improvements in blood lipids.

Many other physicians in Houston, Los Angeles, Miami, and San Francisco and other cities are applying anabolic steroid therapy successfully for therapeutically beneficial changes in body composition for their patients with no significant side effects. PoWeR is committed to supplying physicians and patients who are not familiar with anabolic steroids with information about optimal regimens to maximize lean body mass, enhance quality of life and immune response, and minimize potential side effects. The time has come for effective, practical, and economical ways to improve body composition and reverse wasting syndrome.

20
Orthomolecular Nutrition
by Michael Mooney

This section of the book will tell you about nutrition to help improve metabolism so that you can improve your immune response. Good nutrition also helps you prime your metabolism to respond well to exercise and anabolic hormone therapy so that you can optimally increase or maintain your lean body mass and reduce lipodystrophy or prevent it. New data that is currently being collected by several clinicians, including Dr. Jon Kaiser, the author of *Healing HIV*, indicates that optimal orthomolecular nutrition can also improve metabolism in such a way that lower doses of standard AIDS medications will produce better reductions in viral load and improved T-cell counts because your body is more responsive and your immune system is more able to participate in your defense. Lower doses can mean less toxic effects over time, and more potential to maintain sensitivity to the drugs without developing resistance to the effects of the drugs. Dr. Kaiser has a number of patients who are doing so well using this kind of approach that they are achieving good health using relatively low doses of simple combinations of some of the older antiviral AIDS medications so that they haven't even had to begin using the most powerful AIDS medications, the protease inhibitors. Building your health with natural tools is a perfect complement to optimize the effects of progressive HIV medicine.

To give this chapter an anchorage, I am going to first refer to my father Patrick's SAINTS study, an acronym for Super Nutrition AIDS Information and Nutritional Study that took place in 1993. The study was devised to see if orthomolecular nutrition could benefit people with AIDS. What Patrick did was to provide an orthomolecular diet (I will explain the word orthomolecular in a minute) and supplementation to twenty-five people for two months while he kept track of various measurements and the participants' subjective feelings of their quality of life. This study used some of the same dietary supplements I recommend, but only lasted a short two months. If you are diligent in using the information in this section to address your own nutritional needs over the long term, you could experience even greater success. The dietary suggestions in this section work well as the basis for the best bodybuilding and the best immune health diet, and provide more tools that may help reduce lipodystrophy.

In the SAINTS system, people learned about their own food allergies and how to avoid and reduce the immune burden that food allergies can cause. The single biggest burden on the immune system that everyone is exposed to on a day-to-day basis is thought to be the allergens in the foods we eat. While all healthy foods contain nutrients, they also all generally contain a little bit of what can be considered to be poisons, called "allergens." The people in the SAINTS study were taught how to select and cook a clean, allergy-free whole natural foods diet individually tailored for each person. They also learned about the most effective nutritional supplementation to help enhance metabolism and improve natural immune response, which I will cover later in this chapter.

What is Orthomolecular?

The word "orthomolecular" was coined by a two-time Nobel Prize winner, the late Linus Pauling, in the 1960s when he was exploring the beginnings of nutritional medicine with several other science pioneers. *Ortho* means "right or correct," or in this case, "natural to the human body," and *molecular* means of molecules. In this specific case, it means "natural or right molecules for the biochemical needs of the human body" because the body has been working with these natural ortho-molecules for millions of years. These molecules are simply the same health-giving nutrients we get from food.

Let me put this in perspective by telling you that when my father and I started seriously investigating progressive nutrition in the 1970s, there were only about 300 doctors in the U.S. who practiced some kind of nutritional medicine, and only a handful of scientists, like Dr. Pauling, who were involved with it. Today there are thousands of doctors in the United States, including doctors who work with HIV(+) people, who use some of these nutritional techniques in their practice.

Higher Nutrient Doses Work Better – The Threshold Effect

What these pioneer doctors were doing was creating a foundation for health by using a diet of whole natural foods at the same time that they supplied these ortho-molecules, like vitamins, to help correct and strengthen human metabolism by giving the body specific, usually higher than RDA (recommended daily allowance) level amounts of these

ortho-molecules. This was to make sure that the body did not suffer from any nutrient deficiencies, and so could operate at its best. In some cases they found that giving some people extremely high amounts of these ortho-molecules improved certain disease states. I offer to you the hypothesis that there is a threshold effect for nutrients and that some of the nutrients do not produce as much of an effect in lower doses as they do when they are taken in higher doses. (See also: http://www.supernutritionusa. com/vitamin.safety.doses9-02.pdf)

For instance, recently it was shown that 1,000 mcg. of folic acid significantly reduced colitis and the incidence of precancerous colon cells while 400 mcg. was significantly less effective.[282] Decidedly, 1,000 mcg. is an unnatural super-physiologic amount, many times as much folic acid as you would find in any single natural food. However, when given in this orthomolecular amount, folic acid helps reduce the potential for several medical problems. Folic acid supplementation becomes even more interesting when we realize that supplemental folic acid is absorbed about 40 percent better than folic acid found in foods.[283]

These orthomolecular doctors also attempted to reduce wear and tear on the body by removing specific foods that people were allergic to from their diets. At the same time that orthomolecular nutrition delivers helpful natural molecules and whole foods, it eliminates or reduces problematic molecules, including artificial compounds, toxins, and the allergens that I am going to talk about, to reduce the metabolic burden that any of them might create. What these scientists found was that they could do some amazing things to improve people's health with this approach.

Conventional Western or allopathic medicine tends to use toxic drugs to kill microbes; "drugs to kill bugs." And while this approach is useful in addressing many diseases, orthomolecular doctors were using ortho-molecules and getting better results for some medical problems than they would if they used drugs. What they found was that if they strengthened metabolism by using these ortho-molecules, much of the time the body would become strong enough that it would conquer the bugs and or control them by itself. This is a non-toxic, no side-effect way of getting healthier. This happens because these natural ortho-molecules support healthy immune function and the entire metabolism, while not causing the side effects that a majority of drugs do. So, orthomolecular nutrition gave birth to orthomolecular medicine, which is nutritionally based medicine. Orthomolecular is back to nature, but optimally so, using a scientifically developed understanding of natural biochemistry.

Orthomolecular medicine is a scientific approach to improving metabolism by using optimum nutrition to balance and strengthen it. This holistic approach involves simple components in a logical system.

Whole Food

For your best immune health, the first consideration about food is to try to stay whole and natural. This means to try to avoid any food that is artificial, that is, not in its natural form; but don't drive yourself crazy by being too strict about this too quickly. Ease into it if you have to. The important thing is to make it easy for yourself and take it one step at a time. Try to clean your diet up gradually and consistently and use more natural whole foods when you make your selections at the market or restaurant. You will do a lot to improve your health if you only

do one thing: gradually add more whole natural foods to your diet, as you remove processed or artificially-created foods. But one step at a time, always. There is an old Chinese proverb that basically means revolutions do not produce lasting change, but gradual adjustments do. (Source: *I Ching*: "Ting: The Cauldron")

Fresh Produce

You should take dietary supplements too, but there are as yet undiscovered life-giving nutrients and therapeutic ingredients in vegetables and fruits that show themselves as the variety of colors we see in fresh produce. The produce section of the market is basically a fresh vitamin department and a medicine chest. And, while most foods give you simple nourishment, some like garlic, onions, and ginger have genuine therapeutic effects. Eating the widest variety of fresh produce on a daily basis assures you of getting all the ingredients that nature provides that can help keep your body strong enough to handle bacteria and viruses so that you stay healthy.

Besides the fact that organic produce generally has more nutrient content than non-organic, one reason I recommend organic produce is because the chemicals, like pesticides, that can be found on non-organic produce can negatively impact the immune system. Even if you eat organic produce, always wash your produce well, not only to get the pesticides and chemicals off of the non-organic produce, but to get the microorganisms off of any produce. There are lots of tiny bugs living on the surfaces of fresh produce, and some of them are pretty nasty to a

I caution that while there are a small minority of HIV(+) people who get so healthy using orthomolecular nutrition combined with regular exercise, meditation and other body/mind techniques that they do not have to use drugs, standard HIV medications are necessary for the majority of people living with HIV. For the majority of people with critical illnesses, in general, the best effect is seen with an integrated approach, where optimum natural nutrition and healthy lifestyle techniques are used to complement progressive medical approaches.

compromised immune system, so wash produce well. To be extra sure the bugs are gone, you should wash your produce with one of the mild organic dishwashing liquids that are sold in natural foods stores. There are also produce cleansers like "Healthy Harvest Fruit and Vegetable Rinse" that help remove contaminants, like waxes, and pesticides, while destroying common bacteria and fungus. This is especially important if you have low T cells (below 50). Whether the produce you eat is organic or not though, be sure to eat fresh vegetables and fruits on a daily basis as much as possible.

DIET AND ALLERGENS

Is "Natural" Always Good?

There are components in natural foods that are good for us and some things that are not so good. The good things are nutrients and some of the primary bad things are the allergens that are found in many of the foods we eat. Just as nature has toadstools and tigers that can kill us, so it is with natural food allergens. Reducing exposure to food allergens reduces a powerful burden on the immune system that sometimes has a profound effect. Two common benefits are a significant reduction in diarrhea, and a tremendous increase in energy. Allergens come in a variety of molecular forms, but what they have in common is that they produce a reaction that stresses your immune system, which responds to this reaction and spends energy dealing with it. So, food allergens are something to be avoided. How do we avoid them? There are several methods to detect these allergens, and several ways to handle them once we do.

Four-Day Rotating Diet

One of the easiest ways to handle allergens is to just rotate your foods so that you do not eat from the same food family more than once every four days. With this method, unless you are severely allergic to some food, you will not even have to sleuth out which foods you are actually allergic to. This is called a four-day rotating diet and there are a number of books that tell you all about it. The common allergens that you would rotate or avoid include some of the world's most popular foods: wheat, corn, milk/dairy, bananas, yeast (beer), peanuts, chocolate, tomatoes, citrus, soy, and coffee. Sounds like many peoples' shopping list, doesn't it? The important thing to remember is to rotate your foods so you do not eat the same ones regularly. You benefit in many ways because you end up getting a variety of different kinds of food and a wider variety of nutrients.

How Do You Know What You Are Allergic To?

Do you say to yourself that a symptom like diarrhea is "just because I have AIDS?" Sometimes someone who is HIV(+) will have diarrhea of unknown origin and the standard medical tests will not be able to tell what is causing it, so it is dubbed "HIV enteropathy." This is a classic time to look for hidden food allergies. Food allergies can cause this kind of upset in the gastrointestinal system very easily, without cryptosporidium, or amoebas, or any other pathogen. How do we find out what we are allergic to? The best thing to do is look for cause and effect. This is where the elimination diet can help you find out what you are allergic to.

Food Allergy Rule of Thumb: Look For Cause and Effect

- If I drink milk do I . . . get diarrhea later that day or get mucus right away?
- If I eat wheat do I . . . feel depressed two hours later, or get headaches?
- If eat tomatoes do I . . . get skin rashes the next day?

These are some of the kinds of reactions to food allergens that are common.

Solutions

These are the solutions commonly used to detect food allergies so that you can change your diet accordingly. The easiest is item #1 and the best is item #3.

1. Avoid the most common allergens listed above and rotate your foods. See the Food Allergen Chart.

2. Self-test yourself: Read any book on the subject and follow instructions to self-test for allergens. Books include: *Dr. Mandell's 5-Day Allergy Relief System*; *Do It Yourself Allergy Analysis* by Ludeman, and *Are You Allergic* by Crook. This is a partial list; there are a lot more books at natural food stores. Then, keep a Personal Food Allergy Journal and look for cause and effect. Eliminating foods that are suspected of causing allergies one by one can tell you a lot about what causes your problems.

3. Get professional allergy screening, which is a clinical test procedure that can give you an assessment of your food allergies with less effort on your part. If your doctor does not know how to do this, he or she should be able to refer you to specialists who are geared to do this. Several of the best tests are the Elisa/ACT, functional assessment tests like the liver detoxification panel from Serammune physicians, and the digestive analysis tests, and the intestinal permeability test from Great Smokies Laboratories. Ask your physician, registered dietitian, or certified nutritionist if they know about these tests.

FOOD ALLERGEN CHART

This list presents what are regarded as the most allergenic foods by food group. Individuals will vary in exactly how they react to different foods, as allergenicity depends on many factors, including frequency of exposure to the food, and genetics. If your ancestors evolved eating a given food, there is usually less potential that you are allergic to it. The foods that are most commonly allergenic are listed at the top of the table. Less commonly allergenic ones are at the bottom.

Animal Products	Vegetables	Nuts and Seeds	Fruits	Grains
Egg	Tomato Spinach	Peanut Hazelnut (filbert)	Strawberry Fig Mango Raspberry Orange	Wheat Semolina Bulgar Triticale Spelt
Skim milk	Celery (raw) Carrot (raw) Green pea Beans Cabbage (core)	Walnut Pecan Brazil nut Almond	Apple (raw) Apricot (raw) Peach (raw) Date	Corn

Animal Products	Vegetables	Nuts and Seeds	Fruits	Grains
Shellfish – Crab – Lobster – Prawn/shrimp – Clam – Oyster	Cauliflower Brussels sprouts Green bean	Cocoa bean Chocolate Coconut	Cantaloupe Raisin Pineapple Apple (cooked)	Oats
Goat cheese	Avocado Cabbage (outer leaves)	Cashew Pistachio Macadamia	Cherry Kiwi Plum/prune Apricot (cooked)	Rye/Barley
Cheese	Onions	Legumes – Soy – Dried peas – Lentils – Dried beans – Navy – Pinto – Garbanzo	Loganberry Boysenberry	Rice
Fin fish – Cod – Sole/whitefish – Tuna – Salmon	Celery (cooked) Green/red Peppers		Banana Grape	Quinoa
Ham Pork	Potato Cucumber Lettuce	Sesame seed Pumpkin seed	Grapefruit Lemon Lime	Buckwheat
Chicken Beef	Asparagus Broccoli Beets		Watermelon Currants	Amaranth
Buttermilk Yogurt	Squash	Carob	Peach (cooked/ canned)	Arrowroot

Animal Products	Vegetables	Nuts and Seeds	Fruits	Grains
Wild game – Deer – Elk – Moose – Buffalo	Carrot (cooked) Parsnip Bean sprouts		Cranberry Blackberry Blueberry	Millet
Butter	Turnip Sweet potato Yam		Pear	
Turkey Lamb Rabbit			Rhubarb	

THE COMPONENTS OF WHOLE FOOD

Foods are made up of many different components, some are "micro" or smaller quantity nutrients, like vitamins, and some are "macro" or larger quantity nutrients. The three macro-groups that compose the majority of our diets are carbohydrates, proteins and fats. These three units are the basic materials that fuel our activities and maintain our lean body mass. Selecting the best sources of these three helps to optimize body composition and prevent muscle loss and bodyfat accumulation and dysfunction.

The Best Carbohydrates

Carbohydrates provide our body's main source of quick energy. After carbohydrates are digested and after some processing by the liver, they are released into the bloodstream as a sugar called "glucose" to be delivered to the cells.

Throughout the majority of the last million years of our evolution, the human diet consisted of animal carcasses, some seeds, nuts, and fibrous vegetable-and-fruit carbohydrate sources that are generally nutrient-rich with lots of water, but are not calorie dense, e.g., they typically contained 150 to 450 calories per pound. The majority of these carbohydrate sources are vegetables, leaves, roots, and fruits. Because the vegetable fiber tends to slow down digestion, or a majority of the carbohydrates in these foods are digested relatively slowly, the moderate amount of sugar that is released from these foods doesn't produce profound lasting effects on the elevation of blood sugar. (Note: fruits have carbohydrates that release relatively quickly, but the net amount of carbohydrate calories is still not great.)

It was only about 10,000 years ago, which is not very long ago on the evolutionary scale, that human beings were introduced to higher intakes of grains as carbohydrate sources with the advent of agriculture. The problem with higher intakes of grains is that grains deliver lots of calories (energy), approximately 1,200 to 1,600 calories per pound. Additionally, some grains deliver their sugar energy relatively quickly, especially if the grain is milled, as are breads and pasta. When a large amount of sugar energy is released into the bloodstream it creates a dysfunctional hormonal environment that can ultimately promote several of the diseases that we associate with modern society, including obesity, cardiovascular disease, and diabetes. This hormonal shift also has a profound effect on muscle and fat metabolism, and immune (T cell) function. The key hormone involved in this problem is insulin, which is produced by the pancreas, an organ.

Insulin and Insulin Resistance

As was discussed in the chapter on lipodystrophy, insulin's main job in the body is to promote the delivery of sugar energy as glucose to cells. When a small amount of glucose is delivered into the bloodstream, a small amount of insulin is produced by the pancreas to accompany it. When there is a large amount of glucose, the pancreas works to produce a large amount of insulin to facilitate its delivery so that cells can take in as much glucose as is possible. Extra glucose that cannot be taken in by the cells circulates in the bloodstream, and, under normal circumstances, most of it is soon converted into triglycerides (fat) so that the unused energy can be stored.

The correct amount of healthy carbohydrate sources will provide enough sugar to give a healthy amount of glucose to the cells, but not too much at once, so that levels of glucose and insulin in the bloodstream are not unusually elevated for any long time period. The pancreas works, but it is not overworked trying to keep up with an unusual demand for insulin. However, in modern American society, much of the diet consists not only of large amounts of high calorie carbohydrate sources, such as grains like wheat and corn, but carbohydrates from sweets, which are very concentrated sources of sugar. The net effect that intake of these calorie-dense carbohydrate foods creates is a bloodstream that is occasionally flooded with large amounts of glucose, a pancreas that is overworked, and large amounts of insulin and triglycerides circulating in the bloodstream. Note that excess insulin causes increased production of cholesterol.

Over time, these occasional glucose, triglyceride and insulin floods can cause a decrease in the sensitivity of the cell's response to insulin, which reduces the cell's ability to take in glucose. This is similar to what would happen if you listened to extremely loud rock music, or worked on jet engines frequently over several years; after a while your hearing, which is normally sensitivity to sound, would suffer, and you would become insensitive to noise. Insensitivity to insulin is called insulin resistance, and it is a serious consideration in HIV because we are now seeing it as one of the core components of body fat redistribution syndrome, also known as lipodystrophy, which was addressed earlier.

This is why it is best to select the majority of your carbohydrate intake from slow-releasing carbohydrate sources that do not contain an excessive amount of calories. You will have less potential to experience insulin resistance, and you will find that you gain muscle without fat more easily when your insulin mechanism is healthy.

Carbohydrate Pecking Order

This section presents the suggested pecking order of carbohydrate food sources that shows you which carbohydrate sources support your health without increasing insulin resistance. Best are vegetables in their many forms. Raw or steamed vegetables should be included whenever you eat. They are foundation materials and basically cannot be over-consumed. It is almost impossible to get fat eating vegetables, unless they are cooked in oil. Then come fruits; the sweetest ones should be eaten somewhat sparingly if body fat is a problem, and the best times to eat them are first thing in the morning or right after a workout when insulin sensitivity is high. Bananas are among the fruits to be moderate with if body fat is a problem, because they are among the sweetest, highest calorie per pound of the fruits. Next in the pecking order are beans and peas. These deliver more calories than vegetables, but the carbohydrates release relatively slowly, much more slowly than grains. Next are whole grains, including oatmeal, barley, and rye, which are calorie dense, but contain carbohydrates that, in general, release somewhat slowly. At the very bottom of the pecking order, and the most likely to promote body fat problems, are carbohydrates from grains like wheat and corn. Whole grains are marginally better than processed grains, but when they are milled into flour the difference is not that great. The very worst carbohydrate sources are sweets, like candies, which can deliver as much as 2000 calories per pound.

I suggest that people reduce the use of wheat in general, even whole wheat, especially if the wheat is in milled form, like flour or bread. When wheat is milled, the carbohydrates it contains digest and convert to sugar very quickly. This can produce a quick rise in blood sugar more quickly than white table sugar.[284] The gluten in wheat and some other grains has also been shown to increase the incidence of neuropathy in normal populations.[285]

Try to eat from the first group of slow-release carbohydrate sources most of the time, and if you are relatively healthy, with no lipodystrophy, you can cheat once in a while and have a little milled wheat products or sweets.

My dietitian friends remind me that some HIV(+) people who have weight-loss problems need all the calories they can get, and I agree that this is a sensitive area that requires some delicate balancing, so each person should consider his or her own situation carefully. But remember, if you have a problem with too much bodyfat or bodyfat redistribution, elevated blood glucose, elevated triglycerides or elevated cholesterol, high-calorie starchy carbohydrates from foods like pasta and bread can be your worst enemy.

Timing Meals for Best Muscle Growth

For bodybuilding purposes there is a time when it is advantageous to allow blood sugar to elevate so that insulin helps the muscle-growing process. This means timing meals that contain carbohydrates, and especially simple carbohydrates, for best modulation of natural insulin production to enhance muscle growth. The simplest and best suggestion is to drink a high-carbohydrate, high-protein lowfat or non-fat bodybuilding drink immediately after weight training, as this is the time when a rapid rise in insulin levels will drive the carbohydrates and amino acids into the muscle cells. After the drain of exercise, the body can basically be starved for carbohydrates and amino acids and is primed to transport them into the muscles more efficiently, with less potential for the calories to spill over and be transformed into fat for storage. A rapid rise in insulin to enhance energy delivery into cells at this time is desirable to enhance muscle growth. This after-exercise meal could also be the highest-calorie meal of the day.

Combining Carbohydrates with Protein, Fiber and Fat

If you eat quick-releasing, high-calorie carbohydrates at the same time that you eat protein, fiber or fat, they will slow the digestion of the carbohydrates, which helps to reduce the rise in blood sugar. While this is one way to reduce the problematic effect of high calorie carbohydrates, it is better just to reduce the overall intake of these troublemakers, because eating too many calories is actually probably the greatest promoter of health problems, overall. I underline that eating a combination of high calorie carbohydrates or sweets with fats causes us to gain more body fat than any other combination. (Think ice cream or pizza.) Neither fat nor carbohydrates alone will produce as much of a problem as this combination, so keep this in mind if you want to keep your bodyfat at a healthy low level.

The Glycemic Index of Various Carbohydrates

Most of the time, try to eat below 69 percent on the Glycemic Index below. This scale tells us basically how much a carbohydrate raises blood sugar and upsets insulin balance when eaten by itself. The higher the percentage, the greater the rise in blood sugar. Notice how sweet foods, or foods that release sugar quickly, are at the top. To be clear, in real-world situations carbohydrates are usually combined with fiber, protein, and fat. Combinations tend to blunt the effect that carbohydrates can have on raising blood sugar, and so this table is only a reference point, and not to be taken as gospel. Foods high on this chart, eaten regularly and in quantity, can increase the potential for insulin resistance, diabetes, atherosclerosis, and perhaps lipodystrophy, especially when eaten in quantity. If you do eat them, be sparing.

Sweeteners

Nutrasweet/aspartame is used in most of the top-selling protein powder drink mixes because it replaces sugar as a sweetener so that the drink can give you muscle-building protein without giving you fat-making sugar, and still taste sweet. There are two sides to the aspartame story, though.

People with a genetic disease called phenylketonuria get what amounts to toxic reactions from aspartame. Another small percentage of the population appears to have a tendency toward having phenylketonuria. If you are one of these people, you may get headaches, dizziness, or nervous system problems from aspartame. There have also been numerous reports from the general population to the Food and Drug Administration of reactions to aspartame that resemble poisoning of the nervous system, with symptoms like blindness, dizziness and multiple sclerosis-like effects occurring. Whether aspartame is truly toxic or not is controversial, but I personally avoid this totally unnatural molecule.

If you have bodyfat problems try to minimize sweetening with sugar and honey, or "natural" brown sugar, because all sugary sweeteners can upset the insulin balance.

In 1999 the Food and Drug Administration approved a new sugar substitute called sucralose (Splenda) that tastes like table sugar (sucrose). Sucralose is a "chlorinated" version of sucrose. The chlorination is supposed to prevent it from being metabolized so that it does not deliver calories or raise blood sugar. It appears that as much as 40 percent of sucralose is absorbed, and that it may cause shrinking of the thymus, enlargement of the liver

Glycemic Index Scale

100% – Glucose

80-90% – Honey, fruit juices, corn flakes, carrot juice, instant mashed potatoes or rice, raisins, cream of wheat

70-79% – White bread, white rice, whole wheat bread, pasta, bananas

60-69% – Brown rice, green peas, grapes, yams, oranges

50-59% – Apples, pear, oatmeal, cream of rye

40-49% – Milk, lima beans, navy beans, cherries

30-39% – Lentils

10-29% – Low-fat yogurt (unsweetened), soybeans, peanuts, fructose*

*While fructose is low on this scale, fructose increases cholesterol, promotes insulin resistance, and stores more readily as fat than other sugars. Read food ingredient labels and try to reduce the intake of fructose and high-fructose corn syrup.

and kidneys, kidney stone formation, diarrhea, reduced growth rate, decreased blood count and other problems, including decreased control of diabetes. For those who are HIV(+) the possibility that it causes shrinking of the thymus, the gland that is central to immune function, should be enough reason to avoid using it. Sucralose might just become the most widely used sweetener in the world over the next few years, so it is backed by a trillion dollar industry that has produced data that says that it is safe. Since it is a manufactured molecule, not found in nature, I doubt that it is truly completely safe. For more information, see:

http://www.messengers-of-messiah.org/piper mail/health/2002-June/000208.html

Fats and Oils

There are a number of different kinds of fats. There is motor oil, there is butter, and there are essential fatty acids. The most important oil to keep a Honda running right is not essential fatty acids (EFAs), but if you want to help your body stay healthy, and your immune system keep operating at its best, you had better consider getting these EFAs on a daily basis. They are called "essential" because your body cannot manufacture them, and must obtain them from an outside source, like food or supplements. They are necessary for every critical function in your metabolism including building muscle and fighting infections. EFAs are one of the reasons I do not advocate a super low-fat diet.

I recommend that you read a couple of books on diets that include more healthy fat than the older popular diets used to recommend. Probably the most popular book on the subject is *Mastering The Zone*, by Barry Sears, which is available at most book stores; this is Dr. Sears' second book on the so-called "Zone" diet. I have heard several people who are using protease inhibitors say that the Zone diet was the only thing that caused their elevated cholesterol levels to normalize. Another book that uses the same

Zone-type principles, but is a little easier to follow, is *The Fat-Burning Diet*, by Jay Robb. (Cost: $12.99 plus shipping; to order call: 800-862-8763.) Do not let the title fool you. *The Fat-Burning Diet* could be modified a little and be called the *Fat-Burning, Muscle Building Diet*. Both *The Fat-Burning Diet* and *Mastering the Zone* will help you build muscle, too, if you get enough calories. Both books support a balanced, healthy approach to diet that can help you build muscle and reduce fat. But be careful to eat more calories than they recommend for losing fat if you want to build muscle.

The main point is that since we need EFAs and other fats for health, we should be getting them in our diets from fresh high-quality sources. The diet I am proposing reduces the amount of starchy carbohydrates in the diet, while maintaining a certain amount of healthy fats so that there is a different macronutrient balance than the old high-carbohydrate, high-protein, low-fat diets contained. This means striving to get fatty acids from several fatty acid sources, the least of these are the saturated fats that we find in butter or animal fat. Understand that saturated fats are not the demons we have been led to believe. When we realize that we evolved getting a certain amount of saturated fat from foods in the wild it is only logical that they would have a place in a healthy diet. One recent study showed that dietary saturated fat and monounsaturated fat were associated with healthy testosterone production in humans, while EFAs had no effect.[286] So, it appears that we need a little saturated fat for optimal hormonal health. However, most people get far too much saturated fat, which promotes insulin resistance and perhaps lipodystrophy, and not enough EFAs, which are needed for the health of the cells and the healthy function of the immune system.

The other important kind of fat that we should consciously include in our daily diet is monounsaturated fat, which we get from foods like olive oil. Recent data has shown that monounsaturated fats decrease the risk of certain cancers, and have an anti-inflammatory effect.[287] AIDS is an inflammatory disease, so monounsaturated fat intake logically has a place of importance in AIDS, too.

Fats are also a good source of energy needed for muscle growth. They contain nine calories per gram, compared to only four calories per gram for carbohydrates and protein. *It is much more difficult to gain muscle on a low-fat diet.* Low-fat diets are sometimes necessary for HIV(+) people who have compromised digestive systems, but they are not adequate for optimal muscle growth for HIV(+) people who can digest fats.

Fatty Acid Recommendations

I recommend that you consider supplementing your diet with essential fatty acids as per the recommendations I give in the dietary supplement section. EFAs include the omega-3 and omega-6 fatty acids. Most people get an imbalance of these two by consuming too little omega-3 fats, which have anti-inflammatory properties, and relatively too much omega-6 fats, which tend to promote inflammation when out of balance. To get more omega-3s, eat more fish, including salmon, tuna, sardines, anchovies, mackerel, rainbow trout, and herring. Omega-6s are contained in common vegetable oils, like sunflower, safflower and corn oils. Try to reduce your intake of these.

Studies show a decrease in tumor necrosis factor and IL-1, a catabolic cytokine associated with wasting, with optimal intake of the omega-3 fatty acids that are contained in fish oils.[6]

Oils and Cooking

Olive oil is one of the best oils to cook with. You can also cook with high-oleic sunflower oil, avocado, canola or any oil that is high in monounsaturated fatty acids.

Avoid heating oils like corn and sesame. These oils contain more omega-6 fats, and less monounsaturated fats, so they have a higher potential for spoiling and turning to trans fats, which are bad for the immune system. Try to avoid any intake of these oils when they are not absolutely fresh.

Also, choose oils that are minimally processed. Most of the clear oils in the supermarkets are stripped of some of their natural components, because stripping them makes them more suitable for sitting on store shelves for long periods of time without spoiling. Do not use these stripped oils. Buy natural food brands like "Spectrum Naturals" and "Hain." And when you do cook, do not overheat the oil so that it smokes. Smoking causes the formation of carcinogens, and destroys the beneficial fatty acids.

You can use a small amount of saturated animal fat like butter to cook, as these fats do not have the potential for converting to trans fatty acids like vegetable oils do. In fact, they are in some ways much safer to cook with than most vegetable oils.

For a guide that details the different types of fats in different oils and which oils can be heated, call Spectrum Naturals at 800-995-2705 or 707-778-8900, and ask for a copy of their *Kitchen Guide to Oils.* You can also find this and more information on-line at: www.spectrumorganics.com

---

Important Warning!

HIV(+) individuals should be sure that their digestive system is stable and healthy before increasing the amount of dietary fats. Increases in fats for HIV(+) people with compromised digestion can cause serious problems. Diarrhea tends to worsen on a higher fat diet. But keep in mind that medications like Norvir and Fortovase/Saquinavir need to be taken with higher amounts of fat.

Avoid Margarine, Hydrogenated Fats or Processed Oils

Do your best to avoid processed fats or oils as they have negative effects on cellular health, overall metabolism, and your immune system. Look out for the words "hydrogenated" and "partially-hydrogenated." These kinds of manipulated fats probably do increase the risk of cancer and heart disease. They also weaken healthy cellular immune metabolism, which means that they might increase HIV progression. Lastly, they are also likely to promote lipodystrophy.

Digestion of Fats

You may need digestive enzymes like lipase to help your digestive system break down fats efficiently. If you have a problem with digestion of fats or digestion in general, you might try taking a supplement that contains lipase (fat-digesting enzymes) or mixed digestive enzymes that include lipase to see if this will help.

Protein Pecking Order

Dairy protein fractions, such as caseine (contained in milk curd) and whey, are at the top of the list of proteins that optimally feed muscle growth. The amino acid balances, insulinogenic potential[25] and overall growth factor content add up to one thing: milk proteins were created to make mammals grow bigger. While there is a lot of hoopla related to which dairy protein fractions are best, there is more misinformation than reality in this area.

If you are not allergic to dairy protein, or are lactose intolerant, for best muscle growth, I recommend supplementing your regular food protein intake with a dairy protein powder supplement at 50 to 100 grams per day. In general, dairy proteins might be somewhat better for gaining muscle than egg or soy protein powders. I say this based on personal experience, knowing that the real differences may not be that great if there is enough total protein in the diet. In fact, the idea that any one protein is superior is challenged by a small short-term study by Lowery, Ziegenfuss and Appicelli that was reported in Issue Number 5 of *Peak Training Journal* (Fall 1998). This study showed that when weight-lifting subjects ingested either soy, ion-exchange-filtered whey, gel-filtered whey or caseine, there appeared to be a trend toward a very slight advantage for caseine, but the advantage was calculated to be "significant." This study suffered because of its short length, so more investigation needs to be done to get a clearer picture of what differences there really might be.

One of the things that will probably produce the most noticeable effect on muscle growth is to make sure you take in a lot of quick-digesting protein immediately after working out, along with the critically important carbohydrates, but little, if any, fat. This is the time when the body is primed for anabolic activity,[288 289] so feed it well.

Whey Protein Myths

For simply gaining muscle, any of the quality brand name bodybuilding dairy protein powders, like Jarrow's "American Whey Protein," SportsPharma "Just Whey," Champion's "Pure Whey," Osmo's "Whey," Next Nutrition "Designer Protein," and Solgar's "Whey To Go" are all probably equivalent. I believe that when we are concerned about how much muscle these proteins will help us gain, the differences between the whey products are highly exaggerated. If someone ever did a placebo-controlled, blinded study to examine which whey protein enables more muscle gain, I think that there would probably be no significant differences among the various products. Additionally, a hard look at the scientific literature tells us that in spite of the whey hype in the bodybuilding marketplace, whey is probably not the singularly best protein for building muscles.

Several of the whey companies say in their advertisements that they have a big advantage over another whey product because they are hydrolyzed, or they are filtered in some high-tech way, or they have more glutamine, etc. From the lab tests I have seen, some of these claims are simply false. One set of lab tests of three top whey products showed that none of them were actually hydrolyzed, though they all claimed they were hydrolyzed on their labels and in their ads. Additionally, their glutamine contents were highly exaggerated.

I will admit that I too recommended whey protein for muscle growth previously, and made the mistake of taking whey's superiority for granted based on limited information (not studying this subject thoroughly) and the recommendations of "experts" in the field. The lesson is "do not take anything for granted," and "every expert makes mistakes," usually in not being thorough enough.

Cottage Cheese and Caseine

When the totality of scientific data is considered, the old standard dairy protein called "caseine" appears like it may be a somewhat better muscle-building protein than whey because of two things. Studies show that it is retained in the body better than whey because of physiochemical characteristics specific to caseine,[290] and because caseine has at least 60 percent more L-glutamine than whey. L-glutamine is definitely one of the single most important nutrients if your goal is to grow muscle and prevent its breakdown.

My advice for the simplest, best, muscle-building protein supplementation is to eat cottage cheese, a rich source of caseine and glutamine, and/or use protein powders that contain caseinates. It is also likely that the very best protein for muscle growth would contain casein with a smaller amount of whey – similar to milk's natural balance. (Note: Some HIV(+) people experience more diarrhea when they eat cottage cheese, though.)

Medical-Grade Whey Proteins

For therapeutic protein needs, whey proteins can be specially engineered to help improve their

potential to benefit immune function and reduce diarrhea. Both of these benefits will help you put on muscle weight and be healthier. There are two medical-grade whey protein powders that are manufactured to cause these kinds of beneficial effects, "Immunocal" and "ImmunePro," although the less expensive bodybuilding whey products will produce these effects to some extent, too. What separates Immunocal and ImmunePro from the less expensive wheys is the fact that they are manufactured to have high amounts of specific protein fractions that purposely address medical needs.

1. Immunocal

There are more published studies produced by the people involved in marketing Immunocal than any other protein product, and the data is strong enough that it deserves consideration by HIV(+) people who can afford it. It cost $99 per month but can be found at a discount for about $70, so it is expensive. However, its value is not as a bulk musclebuilding protein, but as a tool to increase glutathione, an antioxidant your body makes that is critically important for immune function and long-term survival. (Glutathione is discussed in the section on dietary supplements.)

One small study showed that over a three-month time period, HIV subjects using Immunocal gained between four and fifteen pounds without anabolic steroids.[291] Immunocal has also been shown to increase tissue glutathione levels and glutathione content in blood mononuclear cells,[292 293 294] because it contains high levels of glutamyl-cysteine, a molecule that contains the amino acids glutamine and cysteine. Immunocal appears to increase glutathione levels much better than the common bodybuilding whey proteins. This is because the manufacturer takes great pains to protect the glutamyl-cysteine from excessive heat or processing that would destroy it. They also provide you with a special plastic blade blender that they say will not denature the glutamyl-cysteine the way a typical metal blade blender could. Denaturing compromises the molecular structure of glutamyl-cysteine. Keep in mind that hydrolyzing destroys glutamyl-cysteine, so whey proteins that are hydrolyzed have significantly less potential to help increase glutathione production.

Several highly successful bodybuilding companies have made claims in their ads about the potential immune-boosting effects of their whey protein products by quoting from publications that specifically studied Immunocal, and not their product. Lab test results I have seen show that several leading whey proteins, including Next Nutrition "Designer Whey Protein," are not equal to Immunocal for glutathione production. It is likely that none of the whey proteins produced by sports nutrition companies will increase glutathione production as much as Immunocal in the same doses.

However, I am not sure that using a greater amount of a less costly bodybuilding whey protein would not produce an effect that is equal to Immunocal, so it might be less costly but just as effective to use a less expensive whey protein. Data shows that some of the bodybuilding proteins increase glutathione production about half as much as the same dose of Immunocal.[292] If Immunocal costs about three to five times as much as a bodybuilding whey product, but only increases glutathione a little over twice as much as the less expensive protein, it might be more cost effective to just use more of the bodybuilding whey product. Maybe, maybe not.

Even so, until recently I was very skeptical of Immunocal's claims of its uniqueness and recommended against it because of its cost and the fact that it is so hard to mix in water. However, a close friend of mine, a very skeptical medical doctor with full-blown AIDS whose viral load was over 500,00, had such good results with Immunocal that I had to re-assess it. While the most advanced AIDS medications have generally failed to help this doctor, he told me that he felt a noticeable difference during the first two weeks of Immunocal use, and gained about five pounds. He said, "The only two things that I have used for my AIDS that really made a difference that I could feel right away were anabolic steroids and Immunocal." He also said that after a few weeks of Immunocal use he did not notice as much, but he still feels better than before he used it. I recommend that people with HIV or AIDS experiment with Immunocal and see if it contributes to your well-being and overall health – if you can afford it.

2. ImmunePro

The other easily accessed medical-grade whey protein worth mention is ImmunePro. I have reason to believe that ImmunePro is superior to Immunocal in several important ways. While Immunocal's glutamyl-cysteine protein fraction's singular benefit is to improve glutathione production inside cells in the body, ImmunePro provides this benefit, but also supplies protein fractions that Immunocal does not provide that affect other critical parts of immune metabolism, including lactoferrin, bovine serum albumin, and immunoglobulins.

Immunoglobulins (Igs) appear to have a therapeutic benefit for reduction of diarrhea because Igs can contribute to local immune function in the intestine.[295] They are employed in the intestine to help the body fight some of the harmful microorganisms that damage the villi in the mucosal lining of the intestine and cause diarrhea and malabsorption of nutrients. ImmunePro also contains significant amounts of lactoferrin, an iron-binding protein that affects antibacterial, anti-inflammatory, and antiviral activities in the body, including anti-HIV effects.[296 297]

ImmunePro is reimbursable in Nevada and in process in New York, and other states, so it should become easily accessible for those who do not have the financial means to afford it. The company offers a 25 percent discount and free shipping to any person living with AIDS, chronic fatigue, multiple sclerosis, or cancer, or is indigent, even if the person has not qualified for Medicaid, or Medicaid will not reimburse them. Ask about it at your favorite pharmacy or buyers club, or call ImmunePro directly at 800-260-3587, or go to www.immunepro.com.

Egg Protein

Next in line in the protein peeking order are egg proteins. The important thing to remember is that whole egg is probably somewhat better than egg white for muscle growth and overall health effect, because the yolk is a rich nutrient source, and its protein content complements the protein in the egg white. Together they are a better source of protein.

Meat Protein

While real food, like meats, often seem to take a backseat to protein powders by the public because of a mindset created by slick advertising, professional bodybuilders and athletes know the value of real food related to muscle growth. If you do not make real food and meat the fundamentals in your diet you will not grow muscle tissue as well. Fish, chicken, turkey and beef are vitally important foods for best muscle growth, not only because of their protein content but because they contain numerous other nutritional components that are important for healthy metabolism. The message is: *eat real food*, then supplement food with protein powder drinks.

Red meat builds blood, and is a superior source of bodybuilding and blood-building nutrients. These include creatine, carnitine, phenylalanine, conjugated linoleic acid (CLA) and heme (blood) iron, the most absorbable form of iron. That may be why some bodybuilding veterans assert that red meat appears to help improve muscle growth and stamina somewhat better than white meats. And meat, in general, is less likely to cause allergic reactions than eggs or dairy proteins, like caseine and whey. The only caution about red meat is that the high amount of saturated fat most commercial red meat contains could promote lipodystrophy because too much saturated fat promotes insulin resistance. So, be moderate about including it in your diet and choose leaner meats if you do. (Ask for New Zealand range-fed beef at your favorite market. It is typically fed on grasses not grains, and the animals roam freely in pastures, so they get exercise. Their meat contains much less fat and much less total saturated fat than domesticated cattle that are force-fed grains, which are not part of their natural diet.)

Important details on meat: cooking kills bacteria in meats. Stewed meat is better for digestion (chicken soup, beef stew). Roasting is okay. Try not to fry, or barbecue with charcoal. Charred foods are associated with increased risk of gastrointestinal system cancers. Any cooking of meat or vegetable protein that causes the formation of a hard outer skin renders the protein that becomes the skin to be much less digestible because it crosslinks the protein. Hair is an example of highly crosslinked protein. Hair is protein, but it is not very digestible.

Try to avoid non-organic meat because of the potential of being exposed to the antibiotics in non-organic meat, which can be immunosuppressive.[298]

Do not go crazy, but when you do have the choice, choose organic foods, and ask for it where you buy your groceries. Consumer demand changes what is sold in stores. I recommend eating leaner meats, but do not stress out by over-avoiding fat. Remember, fat is not altogether bad, but monounsaturated fats are probably best, and some regular intake of polyunsaturated fats from fish, nuts, seeds and vegetables are necessary for the health of the immune system.

Animal Proteins versus Vegetable Proteins

Animal proteins generally create more insulinogenesis than vegetable proteins, because of differences in insulinogenic amino acid content.[299] In this context, insulin can be an important part of the muscle growth mechanism.

Vegetable proteins appear to score lower for building muscle, but should be included in a varied diet for optimal health. The amino acid balances in vegetable proteins do not appear to support muscle growth the way animal sources do,[299] but the new designer soy protein powders, like Supro soy protein, contain amino acid balances that are close to being equal to animal sources. I am skeptical that soy is healthy to eat in large quantities, though, as significant data asserts that large intake of soy protein can promote certain health problems, especially thyroid problems. (For more information, go to: http://www.mercola.com/article/soy/)

Vegetarian Diets

It is very difficult to gain lean muscle weight on a vegetarian diet. In fact, it is almost impossible for most people, especially when they are fighting infections that burn lean body mass. While I know a very few HIV(+) people who can do well adhering to a vegetarian regime, I find that the vast majority cannot do it and keep their lean body mass. Additionally, vegetarian diets increase the potential for anemia because of a lack of blood-building components such as highly absorbable heme iron and vitamin B12. Anemia is already a significant problem for HIV(+) people.

If you do choose a vegetarian diet, your best protein sources are beans, and seeds and nuts. Digestion of nuts and seeds will be improved by soaking them overnight. This helps to reduce the anti-proteolytic enzymes they contain that inhibit digestion of the proteins. If you can eat them without digestive problems, many nuts and seeds are ideal foods in several ways because they contain protein, healthy fat, and complex carbohydrates in a very good balance for overall health. They also make a great snack between meals. However, the amino acid balances in these proteins do not appear to be optimum for best

growth for humans. Maybe that is why people in cultures who rely heavily on nuts and seeds for their protein are usually shorter and smaller than people in other cultures.[301] Again, vegetarian or vegan diets present a challenge to people with HIV or AIDS who need to gain lean body mass for survival. Unless you are vegetarian for ethical reasons consider eating fish.

Protein and Weight Training

Anabolic hormone therapy is much more effective when a high-protein (approximately one gram of protein per pound of bodyweight per day), slightly hyper-caloric (calories above maintenance level) diet is maintained consistently. Note: Higher protein intake is known to be necessary for the anabolic effect of anabolic steroids.[302]

How Much Protein?

One animal study showed that glutathione production decreased when protein intake fell below 20 percent of normal calories, but 40 percent protein intake produced no more glutathione production than 20 percent.[303] I recommend about 25 to 30 percent of the diet as protein for best muscle growth and immune health. This leaves a margin for error for impaired digestion. I generally recommend somewhere around 1 gram of protein per pound of body weight per day while you are trying to gain muscle – if your digestive system, and your liver and kidneys are healthy. I find that less than 3/4 of a gram per pound of body weight oftentimes compromises optimal muscle growth if you are training hard with weights.

These recommendations agree with published data from protein researcher Dr. Peter Lemon, which indicates that hard training weightlifters will do better when protein intake is approximately 0.8 grams per pound of body weight.[304] This amount, 0.8 grams, is more than double the current RDA protein intake for sedentary people, which is 0.36 grams per pound of body weight. I have consistently seen higher protein intake produce better results with bodybuilders and other hard-training athletes over many years. It is also consistent with the dietary protein intake of the U.S. National Weight-Lifting Team in Colorado Springs. Based on the research of the sports scientists who work with the weight-lifting team, the athletes get about 1.25 grams of protein per pound of bodyweight.

If you do eat higher protein, drinking eight to twelve eight-ounce glasses of water per day helps the kidneys do their job.

DIETARY SUPPLEMENTS

When it comes to improving your chances of health and survival, nutrients can be as valuable as drugs in some respects, with a thousand times less potential for toxicity or side effects. As I said, Dr. Jon Kaiser believes that good nutritional support may improve your body's response so that lower doses of drugs work better, which means less overall toxicity. He also asserts that you are less likely to develop resistance to the drugs, so you don't have to switch drugs or drug combinations as often. Nutrients also enhance healthy immune response, and can prime your metabolism for best muscle growth. These are compelling reasons to optimize your nutrient program. How do you do this? Fundamentals first. While there a number of exotic dietary supplements and special foods and herbs that may be very helpful, the most important thing to include in your life are high-potency, complete, daily multivitamins and minerals. These should include all the essential vitamins and minerals, along with the common antioxidants, as they all support optimal immune health.

You definitely need a lot more than the RDA, though, as a number of studies over the last several years have shown that supplementing with higher doses of specific nutrients improves the potential for survival in HIV. For instance, studies on micronutrient mega doses in HIV disease conducted by Dr. Mariana Baum of the University of Miami School of Medicine found that nutrient abnormalities of vitamins B2, B6, B12, A, C, E, and zinc were prevalent in HIV-1 infected men despite dietary nutrient intake at or above the RDA. She also found that HIV(+) people needed six to twenty-five times the RDA levels of essential nutrients to get healthy cellular levels of these nutrients, some of which are correlative with a decrease in infections and increase in survival.[305][315]

In her study, Dr. Baum found that it took about six times the RDA of vitamin B2, ten times the RDA of vitamin B5, twenty-five times the RDA of vitamin B12, ten times the RDA of vitamin A, six times the RDA of vitamin C, six times the RDA of vitamin E, and six times the RDA of zinc to get adequate blood levels of these essential survival nutrients. And, very importantly, no evidence of toxicity was observed at these doses.

Caution: People who are on HIV medications like Crixivan, which greatly burdens the kidneys, should be careful about increasing their protein intake, as this can increase the potential for kidney problems. Ask your doctor if you are taking kidney-toxic medicines, and, if so, only eat a higher protein diet under your doctor's direction. Those who have liver problems need good protein intake for the repair of liver tissue, but should also be careful about higher protein intake, and should also do so only under your doctor's supervision. It is wise to increase your protein intake very slowly over a couple of weeks, so that your digestive system adjusts. This will help to reduce gas, bloating and other gut problems. Avoid dehydrating liquids like alcohol and caffeine, and drink plenty of water.

You Cannot Get All Your Nutrients from Food

I have heard conservative dietitians say that HIV(+) people should try to get all their nutrients from food, but Dr. Baum's data shows that this is impossible. If we consider that it takes about 5 servings of fruits and vegetables just to get the RDA of essential nutrients, then it would take somewhere between 30 and 125 servings of fruits and vegetables per day to get what Dr. Baum's data tells us HIV(+) people need. Fortunately, numerous dietitians who work with HIV(+) people go beyond the outdated conservative approach to nutrition and recommend a progressive approach to supplementing the diet with vitamins.

While the medical community has done great work in learning to control viral replication and increase T cells during the last few years, they are generally still behind the times when it comes to the importance of nutrient supplementation. At a lecture at the Wasting Therapies and AIDS conference in New York several years ago, one well-known doctor told 400 HIV(+) people that, "Unless your T cells are below 500, you don't need to take multivitamins." Research shows that this is simply wrong. It has been clearly demonstrated that taking multivitamins improves useful immune response.[306] [307] And this is important whether your T cells are 5 or 500.

One six-year study of 296 HIV(+) men completed at the University of California at Berkeley showed that there was a 31 percent reduction in the chance that the subjects would progress to a full-blown AIDS diagnosis if they just took a daily multivitamin.[308] Doesn't this make it seem like everyone in the world should take a good multivitamin?

Vitamins Help Ritonavir Go Down

HIV nutrient specialists Dr. Jon Kaiser, Charlie Smigelski (Harvard dietician), and Dr. Lark Lands assert that building health with dietary supplements can improve the tolerance and response to AIDS medications. At the 38th ICAAC Conference, Gatti (Abstract A-75) reported that people who took Ritonavir with pre-existing nutrient deficiencies (Vitamins C, E, B12, folic acid, beta carotene), were over twice as likely to be unable to tolerate Ritonavir (58 percent vs 27 percent); those who took vitamin supplements were over twice as likely to respond to Ritonavir (69 percent vs 32 percent); and the vitamin-takers had less Ritonavir-induced nausea, vomiting and diarrhea.

Vitamins, Minerals, and Antioxidants with Muscle

Numerous studies show that optimal intake of specific vitamins or nutrients correlate with your best survival. Do not settle for low-dosage, "Centrum"-brand-type vitamin or nutrient levels. Centrum does not even contain the RDA of all the essential vitamins and minerals, and the RDA is barely adequate for healthy people who have no health problems. Even then it is not optimal; the RDA will only supply a fraction of what you need. Get multivitamins with some muscle – they will help you stay alive and healthy.

Complete Daily Vitamins

For years I have recommended my father's very high-potency daily vitamin formula called the "SuperNutrition Opti-Pack" (complete daily vitamins, minerals, and antioxidants) as the most powerful and most cost effective foundation for a daily nutrient program. However, the newest SuperNutrition brand formula called "The Super Blend" may be even better with even more antioxidants than the Opti-Pack. I attest that these two formulas are the best multivitamin values in the world, per penny per milligram. This is not just hype; this can be verified by adding up the costs of the nutrients they contain and comparing them to other multivitamin formulas. To get charts that compare them to other popular formulas, call 800-262-2116 or 510-

446-7980. Both formulas have superior levels of many of the nutrients I suggest (see below), along with generous amounts of antioxidants. There are a number of other great vitamin formulas on the market that can serve the HIV(+) person well; the Jarrow Pack and the AMNI Added Protection III are two of the best. But no other formula gives you as much for your money as the Opti-Pack or the Super Blend.

It is important to emphasize that some of the multivitamin products that are marketed to the HIV community give you relatively small doses of very important nutrients, yet cost a lot more per milligram than the Opti-Pack, the Super Blend, the Jarrow Pack, or the AMNI Added Protection III. The Opti-Pack and the Super Blend are available at buyers clubs and health food stores. Call: 800-262-2116 for more information.

Vitamin Safety

While spokespeople from organizations with questionable agendas, including the United States Food and Drug Administration, have made erroneous statements that vitamins can be "as dangerous as drugs," a little bit of research proves that this is not true. For instance, the first eight annual reports of the American Association of Poison Control Centers, which collected statistics from issues of the *American Journal of Emergency Medicine*, show that during the first ten-year reporting period of the seventy-two poison control stations there was no documentation of a death being caused by a vitamin, but there were 2,556 deaths attributed to over-the-counter medicines like aspirin, and more than 1,000,000 deaths from prescription drugs during the same time period. Vitamins will never be as dangerous as drugs.

For more information about vitamin/mineral safety, toxicity and optimal dosing, read a paper I wrote at http://www.supernutritionusa.com/vitamin.safety.doses9-02.pdf

Misunderstandings about Nutrient Absorption Can Cost You Money

Most claims about one type of a given nutrient being superior to another type are highly exaggerated. For instance, claims about the more expensive forms of calcium, like calcium citrate or "food-grown-type" calcium, being superior to calcium carbonate as sources of calcium are highly exaggerated or without merit. See: http://www.supernutritionusa.com/calcium2b2002.pdf.

Claims that "food-grown-type" nutrients or "food-based" vitamins and minerals absorb better or are more effective than USP-type nutrients are not supported by science. To read about this, go to

http://www.supernutritionusa.com/food.grwn2001.pdf Also see:

http://www.medibolics.com/FoodgrowntypeCoQ10.htm Be skeptical of nutrient absorption claims and high priced products. Money saved can be used to buy other nutrients in the potencies you need.

Nutrient Tests

For optimal effects on improving your health while reducing any potential for negative effects caused by having too much of a given nutrient, ask your doctor to test the nutrient levels in your body. These tests include the comprehensive mineral analysis from Balco Labs (800-777-7122), or the vitamin analysis from SpectraCell Labs (800-227-5227). Ask your doctor about these and other nutrient analysis tests. Taking them will help you know what vitamins and minerals you need to take in higher amounts and help you determine what is safe for you. While it might seem like a good idea to take high levels of all the nutrients because they are generally very safe, you might have an unusual problem with a few of the nutrients that have more potential for toxicity, such as Vitamin B6. For instance, one HIV(+) man who has suffered from neuropathy found through testing that his body was storing very high levels of vitamin B6 (probably because of compromised liver function). While vitamin B6 supplementation can help to reduce neuropathy, having too much of it can promote neuropathy. Supplementing with the nutrients that will help to correct deficiencies can decrease your chances of suffering from infections caused by a weakened immune system, but determining if there are any nutrients that you should not take can be important.

Basic Daily Vitamin and Nutrient Plan

This is a quick-look plan for a simple, effective, dietary supplement program for the person who is on a budget but wants to cover a very broad range of some of the most important nutrients.

These nutrients should be taken three times per day:

Complete multivitamin – 100 mg. B-complex including vitamin B6 with each meal.

Complete multimineral – the daily total equals 1,000 mg. calcium, 600 mg. magnesium, 200 mcg. selenium, 200 mcg. chromium, 30 mg. zinc, with all the other minerals.

Antioxidants – 1,000 to 2,000 mg. of vitamin C and 400 IU of vitamin E per meal.

N-acetyl cysteine – 500 mg. per meal.

Acidophilus as a powder or capsules, as the label indicates.

Glutamine – with each meal, 1 teaspoon (3 grams) for basic maintenance, up to 1 heaping tablespoon (12 grams) when there is weight loss or illness.

EPA fish oil capsules – 2 per meal.

Alpha lipoic acid – 50 to 100 mg. per meal.

coenzyme Q10 – 30 mg. per meal. (Co-Q10 is costly, though.)

Carnitine – 500 mg. per meal (Ask your doctor for a prescription for Carnitor, the prescription version of carnitine, to save money.)

More Than Once A Day

Notice that this plan says "with each meal." Even if you cannot be disciplined enough to take your daily nutrients three times per day, try to divide the total amount and take them twice per day. It is important to spread your nutrients out throughout the day rather than take them all at one meal because most nutrients only stay in the blood for a few hours. So try to take them in divided doses to keep blood levels relatively constant for optimal effect.

Take Vitamins with Meals

Taking most nutrients after you eat some food improves absorption for two reasons. First, smelling food and chewing and eating stimulate the secretion of gastric juices and enzymes that improve digestion and absorption. Second, having some food mass in your gastrointestinal system slows the movement of the nutrients down so that they do not pass through rapidly without the tablets being broken for absorption.

An Optimal Plan

You can go further, with a daily nutrient program that is optimum, if your budget allows. Here are the optimal daily doses of vitamins, minerals, and other supplements that I recommend for people with HIV. The doses may be high relative to the recommendations of people who are more conservative than I. However, the published medical literature shows that the doses I suggest are not considered to be toxic by conservative organizations such as the National Academy of Sciences, and may be much more beneficial than lower doses for HIV(+) people. Many of these nutrients are contained in sufficient levels in the SuperNutrition Opti-Pack and the Super Blend, but for optimal health it is wise to use one of these vitamin formulas as a foundation and add booster levels of some of the most important nutrients.

The *italicized statements* delineate the nutrients known to reduce HIV progression and increase the potential for survival. Items are not listed in order of importance.

Again, the nutrients that should be taken three times per day, if possible.

Vitamins

Vitamin B complex –100 mg. with each meal or three times per day. B1 and B2 can decrease mitochondrial toxicity that is associated with lipodystrophy. B-vitamins are necessary for energy metabolism and several B vitamins have been correlated to *increased survival.*

Vitamin B6 – 50 to 100 mg. three times per day should be included in your B-complex supplement. B6 is being used to treat neuropathy in doses up to 400 mg. per day by nutritionally-oriented Dr. Jon Kaiser of San Francisco. Too much B6 can cause neuropathy, so it is wise to have your B6 status measured before high dose supplementation. (Compromised liver function increases the potential for B6 accumulation in the body that produces toxicity.) B6 supplementation can reduce elevated levels of the toxic amino acid metabolite called homocysteine[309] that is associated with increased risk of cardiovascular disease. Therefore, B6 supplementation may have a role in reducing the potential for cardiovascular disease,[310] which is promoted by protease-inhibitor side effects. One HIV study showed that supplementation of 20 to 25 mg. per day produced an improved CD4 to CD8 ratio, and *an average 121-point increase in CD4 T-cell counts over six months.*[311] B6 supplementation has also been associated with reduced depression[312] and *improved survival.*[313]

Vitamin B12 – 100 to 300 mcg. three times per day if taken orally. However, I believe that most HIV(+) people should be given prescriptions so that you can give yourself B12 injections because absorption through the gut is often compromised in HIV(+) people. (Typical injection doses are 1,000 mcg. once per month for healthy people, up to three times per week for people who are ill or highly progressed.) *Cellular B12 levels have been shown to be correlative with improved survival,*[314] *and increased CD4 T-cell counts.*[315] Additionally, B12 deficiency is correlated with decreased mental function in HIV,[316] so it may help AIDS-related dementia. And finally, B12 helps to reduce homocysteine levels in the blood,[317] so it is also one of the nutrients that may help to reduce the potential for cardiovascular disease.

Folic acid – 400 to 1,000 mcg. three times per day. (I take 1,000 mcg. three times per day.) Supports immune function, white and red blood cell counts, and protein metabolism. Folic acid is one of the most powerful nutrients to reduce homocysteine, so it too may reduce the potential for cardiovascular disease.[318] [317] Folic acid also improves states of clinical depression.[319] If you take folic acid you should take vitamin B12, as folic acid can mask a B12 deficiency. There is a chance that folic acid supplementation over about 5,000 mcg. per day may cause increased production of red blood cells, which

Peripheral Neuropathy

While vitamin B6 and the nutrients calcium, magnesium, alpha lipoic acid and acetyl-l-carnitine can each help neuropathy, several Western medical doctors and nurses credibly assert that the most effective treatment for neuropathy is acupuncture. We also have credible reports that one tablespoon of cod liver oil twice per day stops neuropathy for some individuals.

can promote strokes. Consult with your doctor before any use of ultra high doses.

Vitamin A – A good general recommendation for HIV(+) people is 5,000 IU of vitamin A (retinol) per day total, regardless of additional beta carotene intake. Beta carotene does not substitute for vitamin A. Vitamin A has distinct anti-tumor and other activity that beta carotene does not deliver, and beta carotene converts into Vitamin A at only 1/6th the amount in normal healthy people.[320] [321] Because of metabolic problems, however, people living with HIV may convert beta carotene to Vitamin A even less efficiently. Optimal vitamin A status improves insulin sensitivity,[322] so vitamin A is a nutrient that might help reduce lipodystrophy. Vitamin A is also required for healthy testosterone production,[323] and growth hormone production.[324] Vitamin A deficiency increases the chance of mother to child transmission of HIV.[325] *Optimal vitamin A status has been shown to improve chances of survival and correlate with higher CD4 T-cell counts.*[326] Be aaware that vitamin A can be toxic to the liver in very high doses, so people with liver problems should consult with their doctors before increasing their vitamin A dosage. (Conservative estimates of toxic effects begin at about 10,000 IU per day,[327] but studies have investigated much higher doses in different populations and shown surprising safety at very high doses: 25,000 IU[328] to 300,000 IU[329] per day.)

Vitamin C – 1,000 to 3,000 mg. three times per day for maintenance, and up to 20,000 mg. per day when ill. Vitamin C has a bowel-tolerance level effect. This means that when you take more than the amount that your body needs, you will experience gas and then maybe diarrhea. This is basically harmless. Many people find that they can take much more than their normal bowel tolerance level when they are sick, without having diarrhea, as the body appears to use it up at a higher rate during illness. To find the optimum dose when fighting illness, raise the amount you take until you get some gas, then back off a little to a lower dose that causes no problem. Vitamin C has not been shown to be truly toxic at any dose.[330]

Vitamin E – 200 to 800 IU three times per day. This important antioxidant vitamin is the best nutrient to reduce the potential for atherosclerosis caused by protease inhibitors because it inhibits the oxidation of blood cholesterol and triglycerides. If enough vitamin E is present in the blood, elevated cholesterol or triglycerides have much less chance of oxidizing and contributing to atherosclerosis. One study reported that vitamin E supplementation improves T-cell response.[331] Another study showed a decrease in the catabolic cytokine IL-1 with 1,200 IU of daily vitamin E.[332] Optimal vitamin E status also improves insulin sensitivity,[333] so vitamin E is a nutrient that might help reduce some lipodystrophy symptoms. *Studies show that vitamin E is one of the*

Vitamins C and E Reduce Viral Load

A placebo-controlled study of forty-nine subjects over three months using 1,000 mg. of vitamin C combined with 800 IU of vitamin E per day showed reduced oxidative stress, reduced plasma lipid oxidation, and a trend towards reduction in viral load (-0.45-log versus +0.5-log for placebo). The researchers said: "This is worthy of larger clinical trials, especially in HIV(+) people who cannot afford new combination therapies."[335] This has important implications for all HIV(+) people, but especially for people in third-world countries who cannot afford the expensive antiretroviral AIDS medications.

nutrients that is most correlative with reducing HIV progression to AIDS.[331] [334]

Minerals

Calcium – 300 mg. or more three times per day. Take for strong bones, nerve health, and muscle growth itself. Calcium and magnesium are nutrients that Dr. Jon Kaiser recommends to prevent and treat neuropathy. Optimal calcium intake improves insulin sensitivity,[336] so calcium is another nutrient that might help reduce some lipodystrophy symptoms. Calcium supplementation at 500 mg. twice daily can reduce protease inhibitor-induced diarrhea.[337]

Magnesium – 200 mg. or more three times per day. Necessary for bone, heart and nerve health, and muscle growth and strength. Also involved in healthy insulin metabolism, so magnesium supplementation may reduce the potential for some lipodystrophy symptoms.

Zinc – 10 to 30 mg. three times per day. Improves healing and immune function. One poorly designed questionnaire-based study suggested that having too much zinc might decrease survival in HIV.[338] Other studies show: there is a correlation with low zinc status and an increase in bacterial infections;[339] high dose zinc supplementation (200 mg. per day) can reduce the incidence of the deadly lung infection pneumocystis and incidence of candida infections, and cause *an increase in CD4 T cells and body weight;*[291] *and that low zinc status in HIV is associated with increased risk of death.*[24] While there is an upper limit to how much zinc is safe (it can interfere with selenium's beneficial antitumor and antiviral effects), after communicating with leading zinc researchers, I find that the potentially safe upper-dose limit for short term use appears to be approximately 150 mg. per day. Zinc is required for healthy testosterone production,[340] and IGF-1 production.[341] *Zinc can inhibit the activity of several of the herpes viruses,*[342] *and there appears to be an association between herpes and immune destruction in*

HIV.[283] High dose zinc has been shown to significantly reduce cold symptoms.[343] (To fight herpes outbreaks and colds I take high dose zinc or use zinc acetate lozenges myself with great success. I always add 2 mg. of copper per 50 mg. of zinc because copper is required with zinc in the manufacture of a super oxide dismutase, which are important antioxidants that are made in the body.) Zinc is best taken alone before bedtime for optimal absorption. *Nutrition expert Dr. Richard Beach at the University of Miami says that many HIV(+) people need 75 or more mg. of zinc per day, and Dr. Baum's study, as cited earlier, indicated 90 mg. per day was needed to get adequate blood levels for many HIV(+) people.*

While I would not suggest overloading with zinc, poor zinc absorption and increased need for zinc by HIV(+) people makes an optimal level of zinc supplementation very important. (Note: an overload is not well defined, and is very individual.) If a person is ill or is highly progressed, it is possible that he or she will need as much as 90 to 200 mg. of zinc per day. High-dose zinc is generally only advisable for short periods of time such as two weeks, though, and only for specific reasons. Ask your doctor or a certified nutritionist or registered dietitian if you think you might need high doses of zinc, and show them this information because they may not be aware of it. Symptoms of zinc deficiency are poor sense of smell and taste, slow healing, poor quality skin and hair, and low neutrophil counts.

Selenium – 100 to 200 mcg. three times per day. Works with vitamin E, and helps in the generation of glutathione, the body's critically important natural antioxidant. One HIV study found correlations between CD4 T-cell counts, selenium levels, and glutathione levels.[345] *In a study of 125 HIV-infected men and women, Dr. Marianna Baum found that patients with selenium deficiency were 19.9 times more likely to die of AIDS than patients with adequate selenium levels.*[345] She theorizes that the link between selenium and mortality is due to selenium's antioxidant function or action in gene regulation that might actually affect the replication of HIV itself. *"In selenium deficiency the HIV virus reproduces faster,"* she said.

Copper – 2 mg. Necessary for healing, and helps form super oxide dismutase (SOD), an important antioxidant enzyme in the body. If you are taking high dose zinc (more than 40 mg. per day) you may need to take more than 2 mg. of copper, as high dose zinc can induce a copper deficiency. Copper is critical to immune health and antioxidant production in the body. Ask your doctor to test for zinc and copper deficiencies.

Chromium – 300 mcg. three times per day. Chromium supplementation improved insulin sensitivity 40 percent in a study with diabetics without toxicity at 1,000 mcg per day,[346] so chromium is another nutrient that might help reduce some lipodystrophy symptoms. (Chromium's potentially toxic dose is considered to be about 70,000 mcg. per day according to the U.S. Environmental Protection Agency.)

Iron – 18 to 50 mg. A six-year study at the University of California at Berkeley showed that iron intake was highly correlative with reducing progression of HIV to full-blown AIDS, and 54 mg. per day from food and supplements appeared to be about twice as good as 36 mg. to reduce HIV progression.[308] Iron is poorly absorbed in general, so supplementation can be very important for people who are anemic and suffer from low energy. Iron is necessary for the production of carnitine in the body, the health of the red blood cells, immune health, the body's ability to fight bacteria, and energy production.

Iron is an essential nutrient, and the body properly utilizes iron for optimal health when oxidative activity in the body is under control due to an abundance of antioxidants, such as vitamin E and beta carotene, which are derived from a healthy diet and/or dietary supplements. Optimal iron status is required for overall health in early HIV. However,

there is a potential for iron overload in HIV, especially in the more advanced stages,[347] or when antioxidant status in the body is compromised, or when there is insulin resistance.[348] Iron overload can increase the potential for immune problems and increased infections, so it is advisable to ask your doctor to test and monitor body stores of iron by testing serum ferritin in blood tests.

However, serum ferritin, which is the most commonly used method of testing iron stores in the body, may not accurately reflect excess iron stored in the liver, heart, bone marrow, etc., according to Sharon McDonnell, M.D., M.P.H., of the Centers for Disease Control. She says that testing for *transferrin saturation* provides a more accurate indication of this kind of stored iron, especially if it is elevated in more than one test.

For those of you who do include iron in your daily supplementation, there is one form of iron that is considered to be basically nontoxic, even at doses in the thousands of milligrams. This form is called *iron carbonyl*,[349] and it is the form of iron contained in the SuperNutrition and the AMNI vitamin formulas.

Vitamin E Keeps Iron Safe

Studies indicate that iron's potential for oxidative toxicity is greatly reduced by keeping your vitamin E status optimum, with one mouse study showing that high doses of vitamin E totally prevented the lethal dose of iron from killing mice[350] Protect your health; be sure that high dose vitamin E is part of your daily nutrient intake.

Special Antioxidants

Beta carotene and other carotenes like lycopene and lutein. I recommend 12,000 IU of beta carotene. *Optimal intake of beta carotene has been shown to increase CD4 T-cell counts and the chances of survival in HIV.*[338]

Sulfur antioxidant amino acids – Methionine at 300 to 500 mg. three times per day.

Methionine is a precursor that converts to carnitine in the body. N-acetyl cysteine (NAC) 500 to 1,000 mg. three times per day. The common cysteine form L-cysteine can also be taken, and for some purposes, like reducing alcohol toxicity, it may be slightly superior to NAC,[351] but NAC is preferred overall for HIV because NAC appears to increase glutathione production more efficiently.[352] [353] While I have heard people say that L-cysteine can be "toxic," L-cysteine is not toxic if you keep it in its reduced state by taking in extra vitamin C. Just be sure to take about three times as much vitamin C as L-cysteine. *The Herzenberg study showed that high-dose NAC intake (3,200 to 8,000 mg. per day) was associated with increased survival.*[354] It is likely that a lower dose of NAC (1,200 to 2,400 mg) would work just as well if L-glutamine is taken also because either of them alone will increase glutathione production. (See Glutamine section below.) I suggest a dose of one teaspoon of the powdered form of glutamine, one to three times per day for this purpose.

Taking alpha lipoic acid with NAC would also logically increase the effect of NAC, so that a moderate dose of NAC (2,000 mg) may work as well as a higher dose (3,000 to 8,000 mg.). (See alpha lipoic acid [ALA] information below.)

A recent six-month study of 262 HIV(–) men and women showed that taking only 600 mg. of NAC per day helped the immune system so much that the NAC users suffered from the flu only one third as much as those who did not take NAC.[355] Everyone in the world would probably be healthier if we all took NAC.

I emphasize that taking NAC can raise glutathione levels in the body, but taking glutathione itself orally does not, as it is destroyed very quickly after ingestion. Also note that the Herzenberg study states, *"The unnecessary or excessive use of acetaminophen (Tylenol), alcohol, or other drugs known to deplete glutathione should be avoided by HIV-infected individuals."* While an occasional beer or wine may not present that much problem to some people, ideally HIV(+) people would avoid alcohol, especially if they are using liver toxic medications.

Alpha lipoic acid (ALA) – 100 to 300 mg. three times per day. *ALA is perhaps the most important antioxidant for HIV(+) people to take.* It appears to be a nutrient that will be shown to be very effective for reducing damage to the liver for people who are taking liver toxic medications. It is known that ALA helps in the production and recycling of the critically important cellular antioxidant glutathione,[356] so taking ALA causes glutathione in the blood to increase. Alpha lipoic acid also may have the potential to benefit those people who have peripheral neuropathy, as it has been shown to be beneficial to neuropathy caused by diabetes.[357] Finally, it also improves insulin sensitivity, so it also may help to reduce some lipodystrophy symptoms.

coenzyme Q10 (CoQ10) – 30 to 100 mg. three times per day with meals. A super antioxidant and important for immune function, energy metabolism, and heart health. Some HIV(+) people report a tremendous improvement in energy with high dose CoQ10 (300 mg. per day).

Specialty Supplements
Omega-3 and omega-6 fatty acids – Alpha linolenic acid (ALA) becomes EPA (omega-3), and linoleic acid (LA) becomes GLA (omega-6) in the body. Note, many HIV(+) people and some HIV(–) people are deficient in the enzymes in the body that convert ALA and LA into the finished fatty acids, which become prostaglandins in the body. Proper prostaglandin function is necessary for healthy cellular immune function. While one popular source of GLA (omega-6) is evening primrose oil, GLA from borage is more cost effective. The best source of EPA (omega-3) is marine lipids from cold water fish oil capsules. You can also get these by eating fish like salmon, sardines, herring, tuna, mackerel, and rainbow trout.

Flax oil has both omega-3 and omega-6 in a balance that favors omega-3. As noted before, most people do not get enough omega-3 from their diet, but get relatively too much omega-6. Omega-6 tends to increase inflammatory activity in the body when there is not enough omega-3, which is anti-inflammatory. Too much omega-6 might promote the progression of HIV. Try to get more omega-3, but you do need both in balance.

A deficiency of either essential fatty acid could increase AIDS progression, as they are both necessary for healthy, balanced immune function. Get these fatty acids as fresh as possible, as they are delicate and oxidize easily. Oxidized fats harm the immune system.

GLA (from borage) is taken as one capsule two times per day. EPA is taken as two to three capsules three times per day with meals. Or take one tablespoon of fresh refrigerated flax oil two times per day.

Flax oil appears to cause allergic reactions in some people. If you use flax oil, make sure it is fresh, because it is a highly perishable, easily oxidizing oil. It should be kept in the refrigerator, and if it starts to taste bitter, the fatty acids are beginning to go rancid and turn to trans fatty acids, so throw it out and get a fresh bottle. The brand I recommend the most is Barleans.

Carnitine – 1,000 to 2,000 mg. three times per day; or acetyl-L-carnitine, a more efficiently absorbed version of carnitine, at 500 to 1,000 mg. three times per day. The prescription version of carnitine called "Carnitor" is covered by insurance, so you can save money if you can get your doctor to prescribe it. Carnitine is one of the nutrients that can reduce mitochondrial toxicity that is associated with the fat loss in lipodystrophy. Carnitine helps reduce triglyceride levels in the blood and is necessary to carry fats into the mitochondria of the cell to be burned for energy. Hypertriglyceridemia (elevated triglycerides), and cellular energy metabolism problems are common in HIV, and natural production of

the body's carnitine is frequently lower than normal, so everyone who is HIV(+) could probably benefit from taking supplemental carnitine.[358] The decrease in triglycerides can help reduce the potential for atherosclerosis that is being associateed with protease inhibitor use. Low carnitine can also contribute to the loss of muscle tissue. Carnitine is one of the nutrients that is known to help reduce neuropathy and acetyl-L-carnitine deficiency is associated with the peripheral neuropathy that is caused by neurotoxic nucleoside analogs (ddl, ddC, d4T).[359 360] Acetyl-L-carnitine can reduce dementia in Alzheimer's patients.[361] Maybe it will be shown to help with AIDS-related dementia, too. Finally, one study showed that high dose (6,000 mg/day) carnitine infusions increased CD4 T-cell counts.[362]

Acidophilus – Lactobacillus acidophilus and the other friendly bacteria supplements are taken to increase the healthy intestinal bacteria. They help to manu-facture some vitamins, and are critical to the health of the intestines, as they keep the various bacteria in the intestines, like candida albicans, in check. Acidophilus supplementation can help people who have gas and diarrhea. Antibiotics kill acidophilus, so after you have used antibiotics you should take acidophilus every day for a week or so to replenish the acidophilus in your intestines.

One study showed that acidophilus increased the absorption of iron and improved hemoglobin generation, so it appeared to help the body use iron so it can build the red blood cells better.[363]

Acidophilus is best bought in dry form and kept cold. There are lab reports that show little to no live acidophilus in several of the liquid products, so it is advisable that you buy it in capsules or, for the best savings, as a powder.

Digestive Aids – For protein digestion or bloating take pancreatin, pepsin, betaine HCL, and glutamic acid HCL. Hydrochloric acid (HCL) is deficient in the stomach of many HIV(+) people. I have known wasting HIV(+) people who have chronic diarrhea who take as much as 9 grams of betaine or glutamic acid or a combination of both of them with protein meals and enjoy a great reduction in diarrhea. If you produce insufficient gastric acid you will be more prone to developing myobacterium avium complex (MAC) and cytomegalovirus (CMV) in the gut, as lower acid levels in the stomach allow microbes to pass into the gut.

For fat digestion take lipase, a fat-digesting enzyme. Multiple enzyme products like "Megazyme" by Enzymatic Therapy or "Jarrow-zyme" with protease (for protein), lipase (for fat), and amylase (for carbohydrates), may help improve digestion a lot. Enzymatic Therapy's "Protazyme" is specific for protein digestion.

**Chew your food thoroughly.
Chewing increases your internal
enzyme production for better digestion.**

Glandulars – Andrenal, Pituitary, Liver, Thymus – Glandulars may feed the organ systems in the body. Glandulars that may be beneficial include adrenal, thymus, pituitary, liver, and hypothalamus. Glandulars are controversial – mainstream Western medicine does not think they provide any benefit. This may be a result of a lack of clarity about the possible mechanisms of action. Personal experience causes me to believe some glandulars do have effects. However, they are not a highly profitable supplement, so companies will not spend money studying them. We may never see good-quality data that examines them for potential effects. However, some older publications do infer a benefit. For instance, an old article in the *Lancet* in 1952 showed that liver supplementation radically improved stamina and endurance in laboratory animals. Old-time boxing trainers know this and tell boxers to eat liver for endurance. It works very well. Liver is also the best source of supplemental iron, as the iron in it, called "heme iron," absorbs about ten

times better than what is found in dietary supplements. (See the information on iron above.)

A supplement called "BioThymic Protein A" is an example of a glandular extract that is reported to improve thymus function and immune function. BioThymic Protein A is available from natural foods stores and HIV-buyers clubs.

Standardized (Milk Thistle) Extract (silymarin herb) – this important herbal extract is a potent liver protector that may improve protein synthesis in the liver that can help regenerate damaged liver tissue.[364][365][366] Recommended dose: 150 mg. to 300 mg. three times per day. Only buy standardized silymarin extract. As with many herbs, the active ingredients in the herb must be extracted to maximize effectiveness. Raw powdered silymarin in capsules does not do the job. As noted in Chapter 12, about lipodystrophy, silymarin can improve insulin sensitivity, too.

LiverCare (Liv52) at 1,200 mg. twice a day has been widely studied in Europe and works synergistically with milk thistle.

GLUTAMINE – AN IMPORTANT AMINO ACID

Glutamine – 4 grams (1 heaping teaspoon) three times per day for health maintenance, or 12 grams (1 heaping tablespoon) three times per day when ill, losing weight or to build muscle. Do not buy glutamine in capsules as you need higher doses than the capsules can give you.

Glutamine is the one dietary supplement that is truly anabolic and anticatabolic for muscle tissue. Studies show that it cannot only increase muscle protein synthesis (anabolism),[367] but also decrease breakdown (catabolism) of muscle tissue.[368] L-glutamine is essential for the health of the intestinal immune cells called "gut associated lymphoid

L-Glutamine Promotes Gain In Weight and Body Cell Mass in Patients With AIDS

by E. Prang, LCN, C. Stoltz, RD, J. Shabert, MD, MPH, RD

Weight loss commonly occurs with AIDS, and appetite stimulants and anabolic agents have been utilized in an attempt to reverse this catabolic state. Nutritional interventions, which enhance caloric intake, are generally associated with fat and water gain, not enhancement of lean tissue. We evaluated the effect of administering the amino acid l-glutamine to 10 subjects (9 males, 1 female) with non-IV drug related HIV infections. All subjects had weight loss (body weight 90% of ideal) and two had diarrhea (pasty or liquid stool 4 times per day). All received 30-40 grams of l-glutamine per day in divided doses (Cambridge Nutraceuticals, Boston, MA) for at least 12 weeks in this phase 1 open-label trial. Following baseline studies, the patients were evaluated monthly; bodyweight, and bioelectrical impedance assessment were performed (RJL Systems, Clinton, MI). Routine chemistries and hematology obtained during this time were reviewed. The average values for the group are shown in the table below.

No adverse effects were noted. Both subjects with diarrhea had complete resolution of this symptom during the study. Six of the patients continued an additional 6 months of L-glutamine supplementation and gained an additional 0.8 kg over this time period.

L-glutamine, a conditionally essential amino acid, can replete body protein in depleted AIDS patients. The increase in intracellular water which occurs signals protein anabolism as reflected by the increase in body cell mass. Randomized blinded trials are now indicated to confirm these findings, which demonstrate that gain in functioning protein-containing tissue can be achieved by providing this low cost amino acid supplement to AIDS patients.

Comment: Note that the Glutamine not only stopped weight loss, but stopped diarrhea in the two subjects who had it.

N = 10	Before	After	P Value By Paired T-test
Weight (KG)	73.0	75.5	0.02
BodyCell Mass (L)	29.5	30.5	0.037
Total Body Water (L)	44.1	45.3	0.021
Intracellular Water (L)	26.9	27.8	0.039
Extracellular Water (L)	17.2	17.5	NS
Phase Angle	6.5	6.8	0.154

tissue" (GALT).[369] Glutamine is also necessary for the generation and function of T cells.[370 371] And, finally, it is one of the very best supplements to increase production of the liver's detoxifying enzyme, called "glutathione," when the liver is challenged by liver-toxic medications.[372] It is likely that it is even more effective in improving glutathione when combined with 1,200 to 2,400 mg. of N-acetyl cysteine per day.

Those who have diarrhea will likely experience a tremendous reduction in diarrhea by supplementing with 12 grams of glutamine three times per day when diarrhea occurs, then maintaining a dose of 12 or more grams per day. This is because glutamine is critically important for the regeneration of the digestive system intestinal mucous membranes.[373] A study by Prang, that was presented at the International Conference on AIDS Wasting in November of 1997, showed that wasting HIV patients who were given 30 to 40 grams of glutamine per day stopped losing weight and started gaining weight. Additionally, diarrhea stopped in the two patients in the study who had chronic diarrhea.[374] See page 132.

Glutamine Doses Needed

How much L-glutamine should an HIV(+) person use? Many people with diarrhea will need 30 to 50 grams per day for anywhere from a few weeks to several months while intestinal tissue repair is occurring. After that, a maintenance dose might be about 12 grams per day. Look for books about glutamine by Dr. Judy Shabert for detailed information. With very little potential for toxicity, glutamine presents several tremendously important benefits to HIV(+) individuals. Powdered glutamine can be purchased at an affordable price in bulk (by the kilogram) through several of the HIV-buyers clubs.

Anabolic Steroids Can Enhance Glutamine Uptake

Another potential benefit of appropriate anabolic steroid therapy is the improvement in nutrient uptake that they can effect. One study showed that nandrolone decanoate (Deca Durabolin) doubled glutamine and tripled alanine uptake in the gut after surgery.[375]

OVER-THE-COUNTER HORMONES

DHEA (Dehydroepiandrosterone)

I recommend the use of DHEA, a supplement available in health food stores, for continuous replacement supplementation for those who test as having low DHEA production, measured as DHEA-S in blood tests.

DHEA is an adrenal steroid and precursor to testosterone that causes a significant increase in testosterone production in women. For men, the studies show no significant effect on testosterone production[376 377] Women also typically experience a more profound improvement in feelings of well being than men, as DHEA can have a powerful anti-depressive effect.[378]

DHEA has also been shown to have potential as an antitumor/anticancer agent,[379] and it has anti-HIV effects in vitro.[380] One study showed that DHEA levels decreased in HIV(+) people when CD4 T cells were below 500.[382] Most recently, data is accumulating that shows that DHEA's potential beneficial effects against HIV may be caused by a reduction in tumor necrosis factor-a,[381] and an interference with NF-kappa B activation.[382] This means that DHEA replacement supplementation, when shown to be appropriate by lab tests, could possibly slow the progression of HIV disease.[383]

If you are getting the idea that I am suggesting that HIV(+) people should consider supplementing with DHEA, you are right. I also caution that you should have DHEA tests done and work with your doctor to find an optimal replacement dose that is specific for you. DHEA supplementation can increase estrogen in men significantly, so estrogen should be monitored.

Although studies have not yet shown what blood levels are truly optimal for males and females, most doctors test to find a dosage that brings a person into the range that a twenty-five to thirty-ear-old healthy person would have. (Again, dosage is something to work on with your doctor.) If a person suffers from low energy, poor mood, or symptoms typical of a severe androgen hormone deficiency, they may find that they need to use DHEA for several weeks before blood levels reach optimum.[377]

I also have feedback from several men who, having come off steroid cycles and having crashed a few weeks after stopping a cycle, reported experiencing an immediate improvement in state of mind and overall energy level with DHEA supplementation. While HIV (–) men over forty years of age would tend to use DHEA at a dosage of around 50 mg. per day, HIV(+) men appear to sometimes need higher daily doses, from 100 mg. to even 400 mg.

Special Consideration – Women

Women who test as having both low DHEA and low testosterone will experience increases in both by supplementing with DHEA alone. I have also seen women try testosterone replacement creams and feel very uncomfortable. Often, when they switch to DHEA their DHEA and testosterone levels both increase and they feel great. Women should consider that DHEA supplementation by itself may be all they need. Appropriate daily doses for women appear to be between 10 and 100 mg. Women should be especially careful in finding an appropriate dose, as DHEA can cause virilizing effects in women. The first manifestations of virilization from excessive dosing in women are usually oily skin, acne, and/or dark peach fuzz. If any of these are detected, work with your doctor to decrease your dosage or stop any use. These symptoms usually reverse if DHEA

supplementation is stopped immediately.

Cautions

I caution men with prostate problems to only implement DHEA under the supervision of your doctor, as the available data suggests that, while DHEA may have some anticancer effects,[379] it might also promote prostate cancer.[384] While DHEA may inhibit certain types of breast cancer,[381] women with signs of early-stage breast cancer should only use DHEA under a doctor's supervision.

HIV(+) males and females should only use DHEA under your doctor's supervision. It can be quite valuable for HIV(+) people, but it is a hormone, and ideally its use should be monitored.

Bodybuilding Supplements and DHEA

DHEA has been appearing in "kitchen sink" bodybuilding formulas mixed with several other purported testosterone boosters. DHEA is not necessarily a useful addition to these kinds of formulas, as it actually might decrease the effectiveness of products like androstenedione, which is discussed below. This is because DHEA competes for an enzyme (17-beta hydroxysteroid dehydrogenase) that converts androstenedione to testosterone, and so it might decrease the net amount of testosterone produced by this process. It also might cause more estrogen production and estrogenic activity because of its potential to convert to 5-androstenediol.

Androstenedione and Androstenediol

I have also investigated the pro-hormone products androstenedione (ADN) and 4-androstenediol (4-ADL) that are sold over the counter at health food stores and some of the buyers clubs. Pro-hormones are immediate testosterone precursors that are one step closer to testosterone than DHEA. Each of them has a much more profound effect on testosterone production than DHEA for women and men.

Androstenedione decline has been correlated to a decline in CD4 T cells in HIV,[385] so it is remotely possible that androstenedione supplementation might be beneficial to immune metabolism, but this is not known. HIV(+) men are reporting good effects on energy and libido when taking these pro-hormones at a dosage of 50 to 100 mg. two to three times per day, but there is no data that is specific to HIV, or data that confirms that they actually affect muscle growth, or what dosing might actually promote muscle growth. Pro-hormones have the potential to increase hair loss and cause other side effects that are characteristic of testosterone, so they should be viewed as another way to increase testosterone, and not as toys. I do not have any data on safe use for women, but these pro-hormones have potential to cause significant virilizing side effects to women, so I caution against any use by women.

ADs do not require functional testes because they increase testosterone by converting primarily in the liver. This means that they will not help men regain their normal testicular testosterone production after they have used anabolic steroids.

It is believed that the potential value of pro-hormones for HIV(+) men in the forms they are currently available in is not as a true testosterone replacement therapy, but only as a quick boost tonic to be used to help improve feelings of quality of life and libido. They also may have a role for periods of time between steroid cycles to improve energy, mood and libido, and perhaps help maintain lean body mass.

Logically, for pro-hormones to increase muscle growth by increasing testosterone, the increase in testosterone would have to be maintained a majority of the time, as testosterone's anabolic cellular effects take place as a succession of events over several days. An AD product that does not have some time-release mechanism, or is not taken several times per day, may have a quick effect on libido or drive, because some of the neurochemical effects of testosterone can happen in minutes,[386][387] but their effects on muscle growth, which take place as a series of biochemical activities that happen over a period of days, would be compromised if they were only taken once per day.

AD products that contain no agent to slow their release generally deliver a quick peak blood level within the first thirty to ninety minutes and then dissipate within about three to four hours. Several researchers have verified this effect by doing blood tests. AD products that are marketed as time-released are beginning to be sold, and this improvement may make this product more effective if the makers really do use a quality time-release method.

Comparing Androstenedione and Androstenediol

Blood tests I have done and others' blood tests confirm that 4-ADL does appear to raise testosterone more than ADN.

5-Androstenediol

Another pro-hormone called "5-androstenediol" (5-AD) is also being sold by bodybuilding shops, health food stores, and some of the buyers clubs. The 5-AD should convert to testosterone at a lesser rate than 4-ADL, and it has intrinsic estrogenic activity, so it is much less desirable than 4-ADL. Because of its estrogenic effects it also appears that it has more potential to promote enlargement of the prostate. I recommend against its use.

Nor-Androstenedione/diol

Nor-androstenedione or nor-androstenediol convert to nandrolone in the body and may produce an anabolic effect with less potential for side effects like hair loss and acne than the ADs. More than likely though, with high doses any anabolic effect of the nors would be about the same as the similar AD product, but 4-androstenediol may increase physical strength somewhat more, just as testosterone may produce more strength increases than nandrolone once a given blood level is reached.[388]

With proper use of these over-the-counter hormones it may be easier to maintain feelings of quality of life between steroid cycles. They are not, at this time however, substitutes for appropriate testosterone replacement therapy. Again, if you decide to supplement with these hormone products, consider working with your doctor, and have him or her monitor you so that you can learn about any actual positive or negative effects.

OTHER DIETARY SUPPLEMENTS

The following dietary supplements are sold as bodybuilding supplements. Bodybuilding supplements tend to be the most hyped, dishonestly marketed products in the world of dietary supplements, so skepticism is warranted.

Chrysin

Is chrysin effective as an anti-estrogen at reasonable doses? Is it a natural substitute for Arimidex or Nolvadex? Synthetic chemist Patrick Arnold, the man who introduced chrysin to the supplement market, has his doubts. Since I have seen no lab tests that confirm that it works, so do I. I suggest that any manufacturer who makes a chrysin product consider doing appropriate lab tests to verify its effects. Whatever company does publish legitimate lab work to confirm a beneficial effect will be far ahead of the pack of wildcat companies who have no credible data to support the claims that are being made.

Tribulus

Does the herb tribulus terrestris increase testosterone? The one study that asserts this is suspect, so more independent data is required to believe it. It is known to be a Middle European adaptogenic tonic herb, and elite Eastern Bloc athletes do use it for improved recovery, but this does not mean it increases testosterone. Tribulus is appearing in "kitchen sink" bodybuilding formulas with androstenedione. If tribulus does, in fact, cause the testes to produce testosterone, it still would likely do nothing to promote androstenedione's conversion to testosterone, as androstenedione converts primarily in the liver, not the testes. Be wary of products like these if you have a real medical need to increase testosterone, as they probably will not deliver what you need.

Lysophosphatidyl Choline

I advise against the use of androstenedione products (or any products) that contain lysophosphatidyl choline (LPC). It is also known as lysolecithin and Plasmologen, which is being marketed in bodybuilding stores as an absorption aid. LPC can increase intestinal (and other) cell-wall permeability, but intestinal cell walls have very tightly controlled permeability for protective reasons – to keep things out of the body and in the body. Solid data in the medical literature verifys that LPC has the potential to seriously inflame and injure intestinal cells.[389] [390] I have received reports of people experiencing chronic colitis after the use of LPC, and it definitely has the potential to promote food allergies, cardiovascular problems,[391] and other problems related to cellular inflammation.

Creatine Monohydrate

Creatine is perhaps the best supplement available for quick muscular cosmetic effects and strength improvement for both males and females. With creatine usage, muscles become fuller looking in a very short time, and the power of the muscles is enhanced. Dosing of creatine starts with a loading phase, where 30 grams per day is taken for the first five to seven days, after which a maintenance dose of 3 to 5 grams is generally recommended. The truth is that 10 grams per day for maintenance seems to work much better over the long run. It may be true that creatine use actually influences biochemical changes in protein metabolism that affect muscle growth, but this is not proven yet. It does fill the muscle cells with fluid, which is called "cell volumizing," and it does enhance the body's cellular ATP production, which can result in increased strength and power.

Most people find that when they stop continuous use of creatine, they lose water and weight quickly. Still, it can be a useful adjunct to a weight-training program, and can be used effectively during or between steroid cycles to maintain and improve muscular strength.

Caution: Some PoWeR clients have complained about becoming very bloated with creatine. This may be because of a unique problem when creatine is used with some of the kidney-burdening AIDS medications, like Crixivan. Additionally, those who have sensitive gastrointestinal tracts should use creatine with caution as it can cause diarrhea in some people.

RESULTS OF THE 60-DAY SAINTS PROGRAM

I started this chapter by talking about my father's orthomolecular nutrition study undertaken before the introduction of protease inhibitors, so I will finish with a summation of that two-month study. People on an orthmolecular allergy-free diet that was determined for each individual and taking only a part of the supplements I discuss in this chapter experienced the following:

- Although most of the people experienced a slight increase in CD4 and CD8 T cells, the average of the changes was not large enough to be called statistically significant. Feelings of quality of life improved a lot, but did not seem to correlate with T cell changes. (No testosterone or anabolic hormones were used.)

- Initially people experienced an increase in diarrhea, probably because of the introduction of more fiber and fluids from the addition of more vegetables to their diet. However, by the end of the study the subjects reported an average 75 percent reduction in diarrhea, probably because of a reduction in food allergies, and an increase in the general health of their gastrointestinal systems. Note: The subjects did not take high doses of glutamine, which can reduce diarrhea even more.

- Red blood cell values improved for most people. Mean corpuscular volume, hematocrit, and hemoglobin values increased (hemoglobin helps to deliver more oxygen to the cells in your body). This is especially important for overall energy and every aspect of healthy metabolism, including setting the stage for best muscle growth.

- Without an exercise program, their grip-strength, which is a measure of vitality, increased significantly.

- People subjectively felt more energetic, and more upbeat, with less general symptoms.

- Libido increased. Sometimes, but not always, libido means an increase in natural testosterone production, free testosterone, or the body's response to its testosterone, however testosterone was not measured. It may also mean healthier brain chemistry, perhaps via changes in dopamine or serotonin, but this assertion is only speculation.

Conclusions
- Orthomolecular nutrition can improve digestion and reduce AIDS-related diarrhea.
- It can also help your body build healthier red blood cells. This is important for building lean tissue, improving overall health, and giving you the energy to exercise.

- Orthomolecular nutrition can improve grip-strength, feelings of energy, well being, and libido, with a reduction in general symptoms of illness.

- While no significant increase in T cells was found in this short study, it would be interesting to do a longer study, perhaps six or twelve months in duration, because many other long-term studies, like the six-year University of California Abrams study, do show that the intake of various nutrients supports healthy T-cell counts, and a reduction in T-cell decline.[308]

World's Lowest Cost Supplements

You can obtain the most inexpensive dietary supplement program in the world (approximately 75 percent off retail prices) by taking part in my father's SAINTS nutrient study by calling (650) 738-3017. All you have to do is participate in the ongoing part of the study by submitting a copy of your lab work regularly.

HIGHLY RECOMMENDED

To learn more about how specific nutrients can address health problems in HIV, get the Nutritional Therapies pamphlet from Houston Buyers Club by calling 800-350-2392 or 713-520- 5288. Also call DAAIR at 888-951-5433 or 212-725-6994, and ask for their publication, *Preventing and Managing Drug Side Effects and HIV Symptoms.*

21

Pediatric AIDS: Approaches to Managing Wasting
by Michael Mooney

Anabolic Hormones

The use of oxandrolone and human growth hormone (GH) with male and female children has been investigated extensively for stunted-growth children. While work that specifically studies children with HIV/AIDS has not been completed yet, we assume that what has been determined to be effective for stunted-growth children is a good starting point for children with HIV/AIDS-related wasting.

These studies show that oxandrolone may be slightly more effective for growth than GH, but that the net effect of the two is probably a little better than either alone.[392 393 394] If cost is a consideration, oxandrolone is the better choice, as a 25-kilogram male child would require roughly one tablet of oxandrolone per day at a cost of $5.35, or GH at a cost of approximately $27 per day.

Studies show that oxandrolone produces beneficial effects with as little as .05 mg. per kg. per day, and as much as .1 mg. per kg. per day,[393] with a female child likely requiring the smaller dose, and a male child the higher dose.

Oxandrolone has been found to produce slightly better results when combined with GH. The combination studies have shown benefit with GH employed at doses of .03 mg./kg. per day,[395] and .03 mg. three times per week.[393] (Any evidence of tumors would obviate the use of GH.) If the child begins to experience arthralgia (joint pain), the GH dose

should be reduced somewhat to find an acceptable dose. This suggested dose for oxandrolone has been used safely with non-HIV stunted growth children, but it is possible, based on what often happens with adults, that the dose might have to be higher for a child who was highly catabolic and wasting.

No Estrogen-Producing Steroids

Use of anabolic steroids that convert to estrogen such as nandrolone or testosterone is not recommended without an endocrinologist's advice, as estrogen will affect the closure of the epiphysis, so these steroids can stunt long-bone growth.

Protein Nutrition

Data suggests that protein requirements would likely be 0.75 to 1 gram of protein per pound of bodyweight per day for a person with AIDS (child or adult) who is losing lean body mass, as studies suggest that higher protein intake is beneficial when wasting is evident.[396] Again, the use of BIA is suggested to track any changes in body cell mass. The addition of cottage cheese to the diet will provide optimal quality protein for improvements in lean body mass. The casein protein in cottage cheese has high levels of L-glutamine and is an optimal protein for improving nitrogen retention.[397]

As detailed in Chapter 20, *Orthomolecular Nutrition*, the whey protein supplement called

"Immunocal" has been documented in several published studies to contain superior levels of glutamyl/cysteine, a precursor for glutathione production. These studies show that it does increase glutathione and improves immune health and lean body mass in HIV patients.[398][399]

The protein powder supplement called "ImmunePro" does not have significant published data as yet, but it appears to help reduce diarrhea because of its high immunoglobulin content, as immunoglobulins are known to decrease diarrhea by increasing antibody activity in the intestines.[400]

Dietary Supplements

Multivitamin supplementation and the use of the supplements suggested for adults in Chapter 20, *Orthomolecular Nutrition*, would be applicable to children, but on a reduced scale that is consistent with the relative difference in bodyweight. All other dietary supplements that have been correlated to survival for adults are good for children too. Good supplements include a multivitamin/mineral supplement, N-acetyl cysteine, vitamin B-12, and essential fatty acids.

Suggested is the addition of L-glutamine to the child's dietary intake at a daily intake of .066 grams per pound of bodyweight if weight is stable. When wasting is evident, a study by Dr. Judy Shabert suggests that an effective dose could be as high as .2 grams per pound of bodyweight. The daily dose should be divided and given three to five times per day. Powdered L-glutamine, available in cost-efficient bulk packaging, can be added to drinks or formula, and has little taste. High dose L-glutamine use is being shown to stop wasting, increase lean body mass, and stop diarrhea in HIV.

Resistance Exercise

The child should be encouraged to exercise regularly, if possible, with some sort of resistance exercise modality like Thera-bands. Note: resistance training, not aerobic exercise, stimulates lean body mass growth. The exercise techniques described in this book for adults can generally be applied to children; the clinician can develop a child's individual program. Resistance exercise is best performed on alternate days so that there is enough time between sessions for adequate recovery and growth.

22
AIDS and Food Safety

HIV(+) individuals are greatly at risk of serious illness or death from food-borne infections. This problem can certainly be handled, but you must take this issue very seriously and adopt several basic precautions.

Food-borne microorganisms cause tens of millions of cases of intestinal infection each year in the U.S. and around the world. Do not assume there will be no problems with this just because you are in the U.S. or another highly industrialized country. For most healthy people, the distressful vomiting, abdominal cramps, and diarrhea are blessedly short-lived. But in people with weakened immunity, such as those with AIDS, symptoms are often severe and the infections are so difficult to treat that they can be fatal.

Bugs in the Food

The leading cause of bacterial diarrhea in the U.S., *Campylobacter jejuni* bacteria, induces up to 10 percent of all cases. Of the patients infected with this bacterium, about 1 in 1,000 dies. Half of the *C. jejuni* infections are associated with eating or handling chickens. Indeed, surveys show the bacterium contaminates anywhere from 20 to 100 percent of retail raw chickens. So cook your chicken well.

Other prime sources are raw, unpasteurized milk, nonchlorinated water, and red meat. Cross-contamination can occur from using the same cut-ting board to cut up raw chicken and then other foods without cleaning the board in between. Cross-contamination may also occur during storage of foods. This is a major pathway for *Salmonella* into the diet.

The *Salmonella bacterium* is perhaps the second-most-frequent bacterial offender, accounting for about 2 million to 4 million salmonellosis cases annually.

Individuals with AIDS, and possibly late-stage HIV infection, are at least twenty times more likely than other people to become infected with *Salmonella* and six times more likely to develop a blood infection, which can be life-threatening. In late-stage HIV disease, including AIDS, campylobacteriosis and salmonellosis tend to recur and are extremely difficult to treat.

Of the several types of *Listeria* bacteria, the only one responsible for illness in people is *Listeria monocytogenes*. Besides blood stream infection, listeriosis can lead to meningitis (inflammation of the membranes covering the brain and spinal cord) and encephalitis (inflammation of the brain).

The *Listeria* bacteria are found in unpasteurized milk; cold smoked fish, poultry and meat; under-cooked poultry; and certain cheeses, particularly soft-ripened varieties such as brie and camembert. Even vegetables can carry *Listeria* and, once cut, support its growth. A quarter of the estimated 1,600 listeriosis cases each year end in death. AIDS patients are 200 to 300 times more susceptible to listeriosis than the general public.

Hepatitis A can be transmitted by unsanitary food handling or by eating raw or undercooked shellfish harvested from contaminated waters.

One-cell parasites such as *Giardia lamblia*, found mainly in water, also infect HIV(+) individuals and people with AIDS.

The extent to which HIV(+) individuals are more at risk for each of these illnesses is unknown, but some scientists believe that any infection may hasten the progression from less severe HIV disease to AIDS.

Do's and Don'ts

Common-sense precautions in food selection and preparation can significantly lessen the hazard of infection from contaminated food. A cardinal rule is: Any raw animal-derived food must be assumed to be contaminated with harmful microorganisms.

It is very dangerous for high-risk individuals to consume unpasteurized milk or raw or undercooked eggs, poultry, fish, shellfish, or meat.

The following food safety precautions are good advice for anyone, but they are especially important for people whose health is compromised, including people infected with HIV, cancer patients, people with diabetes, transplant recipients, infants, pregnant women, and the elderly. Source: *FDA Consumer*, 1997.

- Check displays, labels, and containers. Look for cleanliness at meat and seafood counters and salad bars. Proximity is important also. Cooked shrimp lying on the same bed of ice as raw fish could be contaminated.
- Buy only Grade A or better eggs. Avoid eggs that are cracked or leaking.
- Do not buy any foods whose "sell by" or "best used by" date has passed.

- Read the label to see whether a food contains raw or undercooked animal-derived ingredients. Caesar salad dressing, for instance, traditionally uses raw eggs.
- Buy only milk and cheeses labeled "pasteurized." Cheese made of raw milk may be sold provided it has been aged for over sixty days. But AIDS patients should avoid this as well.
- Keep groceries safe. Put raw seafood, poultry, and meat in plastic bags so drippings cannot contaminate other foods in the shopping cart or bag.
- Take groceries directly home and refrigerate cold foods. Hot foods from the deli should be eaten, kept hotter than 60° Celsius (140° Fahrenheit), or refrigerated right away. Leaving foods unrefrigerated for even a few hours fosters bacterial growth.
- Store eggs in their original carton in the main section of the refrigerator. Do not put them in the egg section of the door because the temperature there is higher.
- Be meticulously clean. Wash hands, utensils, counters, and cutting surfaces with hot soapy water between preparation of different foods, particularly after handling raw eggs, meat, poultry, or fish. In other words, wash repeatedly during meal preparation to avoid cross-contamination.
- Use glass cutting boards rather than wooden ones, which are difficult or impossible to clean adequately.
- Be sure to disassemble and thoroughly wash the meat grinder and blender after grinding raw meat or poultry or blending eggs or vegetables.
- Wash fresh fruits and vegetables with water, using a brush if appropriate.
- Protect yourself with a plastic sealing bandage or plastic gloves if a hand has a cut or open sore, for wounds are easy entry points to the body for bacteria when handling raw meat, poultry, or fish.

- Promptly refrigerate or cook foods, including vegetables, after you cut them up. Bacteria can grow at temperatures above 4° C (40° F) and below 60° C (140° F), so temperature is vital in keeping food safe. Using a thermometer, periodically check to make sure the temperature of your refrigerator is below 4° C (40° F) and the temperature of your freezer is no higher than minus 18° C (0° F).
- Follow the recipe for seafood, but do not undercook it. Avoid lightly steamed mussels and snails, for instance. Fish should be flaky, not rubbery, when cut. Never eat oysters on the half shell, raw clams, sushi, or sashimi.
- Cook eggs thoroughly until both the yolk and white are firm, not runny.
- Reheat food or heat partially cooked foods all the way through to at least 74° C (165° F).
- When cooking meat, follow the recipe's time and check temperature requirements, and check with a meat thermometer. Cook beef and lamb to at least 60° C (140° F), pork to 66° C (150° F), and poultry to 74° C (165° F). Use a meat thermometer to ensure complete cooking.
- When using a microwave, observe the recipe's cooking time and directions about turning the dish.
- When using a barbecue grill, precook meat and poultry. Refrigerate leftovers in covered containers to avoid cross-contamination.

- Divide hot foods into small portions for quick cooling, and allow room for circulation around containers to prevent the refrigerator or freezer temperature from rising.
- If food looks or smells suspicious, throw it out.
- Take charge when dining out. As at home, do not eat uncooked animal-derived dishes, such as steak tartar, sushi, raw oysters, Hollandaise sauce, and homemade mayonnaise, eggnog, or ice cream. If you do not know what is in a particular dish, ask. Send back undercooked food – poultry, for instance – that is even slightly pink.
- When ordering eggs, specify that scrambled eggs be dry and that fried eggs be well cooked on both sides. The runnier the yolk, the higher the risk.
- Be extra careful during foreign travel. Check with your doctor before traveling to a foreign country. Do not buy food from street vendors. Avoid salads and raw vegetables; peel your own fruit; and only eat cooked food that is still hot. Drink only boiled or distilled or reverse osmosis bottled water and only use ice cubes made from boiled water.
- A consumer or physician who believes an episode of diarrhea is related to a particular food or restaurant should tell the local health department or nearest FDA office. Such reporting can help others avoid the same illness.

23

Stop the Runs before They Run You Down

by Nelson Vergel

Diarrhea is one of the most common complaints of people taking protease inhibitors (Norvir and Viracept in particular). In my experience with PoWeR clients, the number one reason for failure to gain lean body mass while on an anabolic program has been diarrhea. This frustrating problem can destroy a person's health and quality of life if not diagnosed and treated proactively. So, what can you do while your doctor is trying to find the cause of your diarrhea? There are many dietary considerations that you should know about which will make your life more bearable while you are experiencing this common problem.

According to Peter Anton, M.D., a gastroenterologist and researcher at UCLA School of Medicine, 50 to 70 percent of HIV(+) individuals will, at some point, have recurrent diarrhea. Because diarrhea is usually caused by a variety of factors working together (infections, food problems, food allergies, drug side effects and/or other causes), aggressive diagnosis and treatment are crucial.

Bacterial Infections and Other Causes

It is very important to rule out infectious causes, so it is necessary to obtain analyses of three separate stool samples collected at approximately the same time on three successive days. Cultures need to be ordered for parasites and their ova (eggs) (usually abbreviated as O/P), and for typical bacterial pathogens (often called "culture and sensitivity" or "C & S"). Some labs that process samples from large immunocompromised populations automatically include specific investigations for *Cryptosporidia*, *Microsporidia*, *Isospora*, *Cyclospora* and *Giardia* (a common parasite). Other laboratories do not, so it is important for physicians to specifically request these tests.

Other causes of diarrhea are:

- Bacterial Overgrowth – Colonic bacteria sometimes travel to the relatively sterile small intestine, triggering diarrhea. A lactulose breath analyzer test can help diagnose this condition.

- Functional Bowel Disease – Not uncommon in HIV(+) people, this condition can cause rapid movement of liquids from the stomach through the intestines, resulting in diarrhea, along with gurgling, bloating, increased gas, feelings of urgency, and/or incomplete evacuation with bowel movements. The use of regular and slowly-increasing doses of fiber (to help absorb the extra liquid and give more bulk to the stool) can help. Since this might be a factor, Dr. Anton recommends that one teaspoon of soluble fiber be consumed nightly, slowly increasing that amount weekly until the bowel frequency has slowed. A diet high in soluble fiber could also help.

- HIV Effects – Diarrhea may be secondary to the effects of HIV in the intestines. We often see diarrhea improve in people with AIDS when their previously high viral loads are reduced to undetectable levels.

For further diagnosis, Dr. Anton recommends that an endoscopic evaluation, at least of the lower colon, be made. A more thorough evaluation to rule out infections would also include an upper endoscopy, something he strongly recommends if neither the above suggestions nor time result in improvement.

Recommended also is a stool analysis, available with a prescription from your doctor, from Great Smokies Lab (800-522-4762). Ask your doctor for the three-day test that includes testing for parasites.

Dr. Lark Lands, one of America's top HIV nutrition experts, emphasizes that care must be taken in choosing foods and fluids, since the wrong kinds can make diarrhea worse. She includes these foods:

- High-fat foods – Fat intolerance is a major cause of diarrhea; reducing fatty foods often results in substantial improvement.
- Dairy products – Lactose intolerance is a frequent contributor to diarrhea and gas.
- Hot, spicy foods – These can exacerbate diarrhea.
- Acidic fruits – oranges, grapefruits, and pineapples – and their juices. Limiting these can help reduce the stinging that makes diarrhea especially miserable.
- Sugar – This sweetener will pull water from your system, the opposite of what you want if you have diarrhea.
- Foods high in insoluble fiber – These increase the speed at which food travels through the intestines. Included are wheat bran, whole wheat products, popcorn, nuts, seeds, potato

skins, corn, and a high intake of raw fruits and vegetables (especially their peels).

Helpful Foods

By contrast, foods that contain soluble fiber will often bring considerable improvement. They absorb water and expand, binding together the intestine's contents and slowing the passage of food. Included are fruits such as peeled apples or applesauce, peeled pears, apricots, peaches, plums, grapes, berries, melons, nectarines, prunes, and bananas, and such grain products as white rice, oatmeal, oat bran, and barley.

White rice and white bread, although lacking the higher levels of nutrients found in their whole-food counterparts, and thus not generally recommended for a healthful diet, may be temporarily useful as sources of calories that will not irritate the intestines. Mashed skinless potatoes are also non-irritating calorie contributors.

Dr. Lands also recommends the "BRAT diet" for those with serious diarrhea who can find little that is tolerable. Every hour or so, eat small servings of Banana (one soft one), boiled white Rice (one-half cup), Applesauce (one-half cup) and dry white Toast (one slice). If plain white rice becomes boring, add flavor by cooking it with a beef or chicken bouillon cube and/or with flavorful herbs like bay leaf, dill weed, basil, or oregano. You could also add garlic powder or small amounts of soy or tomato sauce. Note that in some versions, the BRAT diet has an additional T, for tea. But since caffeine can exacerbate diarrhea, stick to a caffeine-free herbal variety.

No Flare-up Foods

Dr. James Scala, author of the book *Eating Right for a Bad Gut*, performed a survey among diarrhea sufferers. He tried to separate the foods into familiar groups that seem to make life better for folks with diarrhea. That is what led him to prepare a list of foods that most people could eat with no discomfort.

He emphasizes that everyone cannot eat all of them and some people need to eat almost any food in moderation. The following listing shows that there are many foods to choose from. Foods are given by category with notes and pertinent facts about preparation.

- Cereal: Oatmeal, Cream of Wheat, corn flakes, Bran Flakes, Malt O Meal, Special K, Product 19, and Cheerios. There is a clear avoidance of hard fiber (fiber matrix) wheat cereals.
- Dairy Products: Lactaid milk (many people use Lactaid milk sparingly), yogurt, aged cheese, cottage, and soft cheese.
- Eggs: Some people have to avoid eggs because they can be highly allergenic.
- Beef: Lean beef either as stew, roast, or steak, or ground and broiled or roasted. No frying.
- Other Meat: Lean ham, carefully trimmed pork, and trimmed lamb. Emphasis is always put on lean and trimmed.
- Fish: Fish is universally accepted. Fish that swim are called fin fish: They include tuna, swordfish, salmon, halibut, flounder and snapper. Preparation includes broiling, poaching, or baking. No fried fish!
- Poultry: White meat of poultry with two provisions: the skin must be removed and the meat cannot be fried and breaded. Some people need to avoid dark poultry meat. Stewed, roasted, broiled, or grilled poultry is fine, but never fried.
- Skin These Vegetables: Carrots, squash, tomatoes, cucumbers, celery and jicama. Remove skin and cook these vegetables until they are soft.
- Vegetables with Skin: Broccoli, cauliflower, brussels sprouts, asparagus, all string beans, and peas. These vegetables must be cooked well by boiling. Steaming is acceptable for some folks, but the vegetables must be steamed until soft.

- Beans: Some beans can simply be boiled. These include limas, navy beans, chickpeas, and lentils. Other beans, such as black, pinto, kidney, and red beans, must be cooked almost to a mush. Some people can eat canned baked beans. Be careful if gas is a problem (you may want to use "Beano," a product that reduces flatulence. Beano can be found in grocery stores, or health-food stores).
- Leafy Vegetables: Avoid leafy salads when there is diarrhea. Spinach is all right for most people when boiled or steamed well. Cabbage, if well cooked, is acceptable to a few people, but most insist they must avoid it at all costs (lots of gas!).
- Potatoes: Potatoes are always eaten without the skin. Eat them baked, boiled, or mashed. Sweet potatoes and yams are fine if well cooked and peeled.
- Fruits: It seems that most fruit is acceptable – if it is been peeled. Apples, pears, peaches (when peeled), avocados, bananas (if not green), apricots (if fully ripe and peeled), plums (if fully ripe and peeled), strawberries and kiwifruit, canned peaches, plums, pears, apples, oranges, and grapefruit. (Be careful to avoid the fibrous section in grapefruit.)
- Grains: Boiled white and brown rice, pasta, egg noodles, and macaroni. Breads and rolls without seeds, including white, rye, wheat, five-grain, French, and Italian bread. Absolutely no seeds of any type: sesame, poppy, etc.
- Processed Foods: Try to avoid processed foods, but there are some that can be used: canned fruit, canned applesauce, and baked beans for some people. Pretzels, bagels, and some mildly sweet cookies may be fine. No chocolate chips!
- Beverages: Most people can use fruit juices, and vegetable juices such as tomato and V-8 juice. Specific fruit juices include orange, cranberry, and apple. Some people are allergic to apple juice and citrus juices, though. Tea, caffeine-free

tea, iced and hot, not strong; caffeine-free cola and other carbonated beverages, mineral water and distilled water are also okay.

Supplements

While your doctor is looking for the cause of your diarrhea, there are many things you can supplement your diet to minimize it. Some of the following have been discussed in other sections of the book. They include:

- L-glutamine: This amino acid acts like a fertilizer for your intestinal walls, which are eroded by frequent bowel movements. We have seen good results in our clients who have taken 30-50 grams a day in divided doses. (One heaping tablespoon is 12 grams.)
- Calcium/magnesium supplement: Calcium 1,000 mg. and magnesium 500 mg, twice per day. Shaman Botanicals "SB Formula": www.shamanbotanicals.com
- Digestive enzymes: These can help digest proteins, carbohydrates, and fats, which tend to pass through the digestive track quickly when you are having diarrhea. Good products are made by Jarrow, Enzymatic Therapy, Absorbaid, and Ultrase (prescription) by Scandiapharm.
- Acidophilus: This is the friendly bacteria used to increase the good flora in your gut that competes with bugs that can cause diarrhea. Take it twenty minutes before every meal. Keep acidophilus refrigerated.
- Hydrating drinks: Drink lots of distilled, reverse osmosis or preboiled water, or soups, to keep yourself hydrated during bouts of diarrhea. Dehydration will zap your energy, and will cause you to lose electrolytes. Do not drink sugar based or caffeinated drinks.
- Psyllium: Provides bulk fiber and absorbs water. Contained in Metamucyl. Do not take two hours before or one hour after taking medications or vitamins because psyllium can bind them and stop their absorption.
- Electrolyte supplements: Replacing electrolytes can be critical to recovery. Scientifically designed electrolyte formulas are SuperNutrition "Super C" (from health food stores and buyer's clubs), and "Pedialyte" (from drug stores). Super C tastes like lemon. Pedialyte does not taste good.
- Growth hormone: As mentioned before, growth hormone may help reduce diarrhea and improve the health of the intestines, but again, to reduce the potential for side effects, find the lowest replacement dose that gets the desired effect. Usually this will be between 0.5 mg. and 3 mg. per day.
- Flagyl: One of the most commonly used prescription medications for parasites. Talk to your doctor.

For more information about diarrhea, you can buy Dr. Lark Land's book at www.larklands.net

Getting Started – What to Do before You Start the PoWeR Program

by Nelson Vergel

Read this book carefully. Learn about anabolic hormones, nutrition, supplements, and the exercise aspects of the program. Get a baseline bioelectrical impedance analysis (BIA) done to determine your body composition. Get it done again every three months after that. Call the largest HIV/AIDS organization near you and ask them for a referral to a nutritionist or dietitian. They usually have access to BIA and nutritional software that can give you some guidelines. Call RJL at 800-790-0205 and ask them who does BIA in your city. (RJL has this information as they sell the machine to doctors, institutions, and dietitians.) A list is also viewable at http://www.medibolics.com/BIAcontacts.htm.

Call one of the HIV buyers clubs to **order a high-potency vitamin product.** (The best buys and the best formulas are the SuperNutrition "Opti-Pack" and the SuperNutrition "Super Blend".) If you need extra protein, we suggest that you get a protein powder supplement.

For those of you who wish to participate in the use of anabolic steroids, you are encouraged to **enroll your own physician**. Present the PoWeR Anabolic Hormone Guidelines contained in this book to your physician. If your physician will not prescribe steroids, be aware that there are a number of physicians that will prescribe anabolic steroids for wasting due to HIV disease. Call the Houston Buyers Club at 800-350-2392 for a referral to a doctor in your area.

Get a testosterone and a "free" testosterone blood test before starting steroid use.

The prescription for the PoWeR cycle (testosterone + nandrolone) should include nandrolone decanoate (Deca-Durabolin – 12 vials of 200 mg./ml, as directed), and testosterone enanthate or cypionate (Depo-Testosterone), 10 cc's, 200 mg./ml, 2 bottles, as directed). To inject this, get at least 50 syringes (23-gauge, 1 inch). Also get vitamin B-12 (30 cc's, 1,000 mcg./ml, 1 vial, 1 or more 1 cc shots per week). To inject this, get at least 24 ultra-fine insulin syringes. Go to www.appliedpharmacyrx.com (formerly www.gulfsouth.com) if you have to pay cash for these products, since they have very low prices. If your insurance pays for them, have your pharmacy call Watson Pharmaceuticals. Never use the Internet to order anabolics from websites that do not belong to reputable U.S. pharmacies (which require you to mail the prescription), since it is illegal, no matter if you are HIV(+). Never import anabolic steroids either. They are Class III regulated substances and you can go to jail for that crime.

Ask your doctor or his/her nurse to teach you to give yourself the injections, or have a doctor or nurse teach your lover or a close friend how to do it correctly. Visit http://www.anabolicsteroidsaccess.com/Injection-procedure.htm for a good procedure on how to inject. The entire PoWeR cycle for three months can cost under $600 if you have to pay for it.

If your testosterone and free testosterone tested as being normal before you started using steroids, which may mean that you do not need to be on permanent testosterone replacement, you will also need to **get the materials that can help restart your natural testosterone production** that are used in the refractory protocol explained on page 92. These include human chorionic gonadotropin (HCG) – 4 to 8 vials of 10,000 USP, injected with ultra-fine syringes; Clomid – 56

of the 50 mg. tablets, and Arimidex – 56 of the 1 mg. tablets. Note that this adds more cost to the cycle.

Join a gym, if you do not already have a membership. Get a workout partner, or if you have the money, get a personal trainer. Follow the exercise recommendations described in Chapter 25, and learn all you can about proper weight training. The YMCA has a scholarship or reduced rate program for people who have a low income or are on disability. For exercise information, go to:

http://www.tbrewi.com/hivfitness/ and
http://www.exrx.net/Lists/Directory .html

Weight Lifting for Maximum Muscle Gains: A Simple but Effective Method
by Michael Mooney

In this section I present a simple yet effective weight-lifting program. You can modify this program after you have gotten your initial muscle gains. You will then be familiar with the new body you are building and how it responds to weight training whether you are using steroids or not. It is best to start this program slowly, then gradually increase intensity over several weeks or months. At the end of this section, I provide details on how to perform the individual exercises correctly so that you get the best results safely. I want to emphasize that this program is suggested as a starting point. After you are familiar with your body, and the exercises, you are invited to experiment with different weight-lifting methods and learn how to modify your program to keep your body growing while you learn to shape your muscles. Elite coaches vary their athletes' programs constantly. Once you get an exercise foundation, you should too.

Safety First!

Always remember, safety first. If something you do in an exercise hurts, stop! Ask for help to figure out what you are doing wrong. Maybe it is just improper form. If you hurt yourself you will hinder your progress because you will not be able to work out!

Make a Commitment to Yourself

First priority is to join a gym if you can afford it. If you spend money on a membership, you will be more likely to stay with it, and consistency is the key to success in any exercise program. Also, try to find someone who is enthusiastic to train with, or get a personal trainer (if you can afford the additional expense). It is easier to stay motivated when you train with someone else who has a vital interest in your mutual success. It is also safer to have someone spot you when you lift heavy weights.

Train Smart – Do Not Overtrain!

Overtraining is probably the most-ignored limiting factor. And it is especially important to avoid overtraining because HIV disease tends to create the same kind of catabolic effect on muscle tissue that overtraining does. Overtraining, which is the same thing as overstressing, can lower immune response and cause the loss of muscle tissue.

Please refer to http://www.exrx.net/Lists/Directory.html
and www.hivfitness.org for more exercise information.

Oftentimes people think that they are not training hard enough, so they increase the number of exercise routines that they perform in the belief that they just need more stimulus! This is one of the biggest errors a person can make – more is not necessarily better! It seems paradoxical that you could work out less and grow more, but this is very often the case.

Any amount of exercise beyond that which is the amount of stimulus necessary to induce optimal muscle growth can be called overtraining. Let me repeat that: exercising more than what the body requires to stimulate it maximally to grow is overtraining. Keep your program simple, work out hard, do just the right amount of exercise to stimulate growth, and you will succeed.

Proper Stimulus

In order to build muscle, the body has to receive a stimulus – a reason – to grow bigger, to achieve what is called hypertrophy. It is really very simple: the body only does what it needs to do – what it is required to do. It is not going to suddenly expand its muscle mass because it anticipates needing more muscles. But if it is challenged to move weight, it will respond by growing. Another way to look at it is if you take any bodybuilder and put him in bed for weeks at a time, he will begin to lose muscle mass – because the body will sense it does not need the extra muscle anymore. You need to deliver the stimulus to provoke muscular growth in the body – and that is what lifting weights does.

Aerobics versus Weight Lifting

Exercise as weight training can improve lean body mass for HIV(+) people without the use of anabolic steroids.[401][402][403] And, while aerobic exercise also can improve overall health if not carried to excess (overtraining), it does not appreciably improve lean body mass, and it can drain some of the limited energy that the body would use to grow muscle. So, when a person is wasting or recovering from illness, aerobics should be eliminated entirely, as it can cause a serious decrease in muscle growth rate and oftentimes a loss of muscle for the person who is metabolically challenged.

Once you have stable, healthy, lean body mass, for fat loss I suggest twenty to thirty minutes of aerobics, three times per week, first thing in the morning before eating breakfast. Doing aerobics with an empty stomach increases fat loss tremendously as the body has used up much of its reserve fuels in sleep, so it will burn fat more efficiently. But if you eat carbohydrates before you do aerobics you will burn the carbohydrates when they get into your bloodstream rather than your own fat. I also recommend doing aerobics on alternate days to weight lifting, as this keeps you from overstressing your metabolism (overtraining).

Set Goals

Create a roadmap that will keep you on track and moving forward by setting reasonable goals for the total increase in muscle mass and body weight you are striving for. Once you get familiar with the amount you are capable of lifting when you start, set goals for the amount of weight you want to be able to lift.

A Workout Journal

Logging your workouts in a journal will help you work out better. The best reason to keep track of your workouts is so that you can see what you are accomplishing. The journal also helps you stay focused so that you can zero in on your goals, that is, you program your mind when you look at black and white. You will also be able to see whether you are gaining at a reasonable rate or see whether you are overtraining; if so you will not be gaining strength, and this will add up to not gaining muscle size. So, keep a journal of your workouts: write down the weight poundage you lift and the amount of repetitions (reps) you lift for each exercise. Then, when you go in to train again the next week, you know what numbers you are trying to better. If you find out that you are weaker than you were the time before, and everything else is in line, you may be training too often. One ready-made, well-designed journal that can help you track your workouts is *The Muscle and Might Training Tracker* by Stuart McRobert, which is available at 509-234-0362, www.hardgainer.com, or by writing to CS Publishing, P.O. Box 1002, Connell, WA 99326.

STARTERS: ONCE-A-WEEK TRAINING

This section is for those who have only recently recovered from illness, or are just getting into weight lifting for the first time. For the first few weeks, until your stamina is up, do only one workout per week. The workout described below is a whole-body workout program. For more descriptions of various exercises get a book, like *Ironman's Ultimate Bodybuilding Encyclopedia*, which details proper form for the full spectrum of resistance exercises. You can order this book by calling 800-447-0008.

Warm-up set (w) weight refers to a set where you use a weight that is about 50 to 60 percent of the heavy weight set that you use. **Heavy (h)** indicates a weight that you are only capable of lifting six to twelve times before you experience momentary muscular failure.

1. Barbell flat bench press – 2 w and 1 h set.
2. Curl-grip pulldowns – 2 w and 1 h set.
3. Squat or seated leg press – 2 w and 1 h set. Squats are a best exercise, but some people have to substitute the leg press because their back or knees will not tolerate squats.

Warm-up sets: employ a poundage that you know you can easily handle for twelve repetitions (reps). Rest for about one minute between sets or longer – until you feel like you have enough energy to go again. Two warm-up sets should be enough to warm all the joints involved without tiring you too much. Then do the heavy set, lifting the weight until you cannot lift it one more time. This is called momentary muscular failure.

Your Personal Best

After you get used to training, it is important to challenge yourself to the best of your own ability and do enough repetitions to get to momentary muscular failure so that you trigger your muscles to grow. Your level of intensity in the beginning will not be as great as it can be later, after you have been lifting for a while. Give yourself time, and allow yourself to grow slowly, but do work to the best of your own ability. You do not have to go to the point of total failure, where you cannot even hold the weight in place to gain muscle. In fact, this is a form of overtraining, and is a technique to be used only on very rare occasions.

Do your "Starter workout" on a day when you feel relatively good. After doing the exercises, you may feel tired and depleted. You should consume a low-fat carbohydrate/protein drink after the workout to replenish glycogen (muscle sugar) and amino acid stores – you will grow much better if you do. A good drink mix is "OSMO Regeneration" (contains no aspartame), which is sold at health food stores and buyers clubs like the Houston Buyers Club, 800-350-2392.

If you find that you feel exhausted during your beginning efforts, pace yourself more carefully and make sure your nutrition and rest are good. You should be getting balanced nutrition (like food!) three to six times a day, and plenty of rest and recovery. Protein drinks can fill in between meals (e.g., three meals with two or three drinks per day). Continue with once-a-week workouts until you find that you feel good enough to workout on a second, non-consecutive day of the week. Then do this same workout twice a week. When you feel good enough to workout three days a week, it is time to start splitting the exercise routine up to work on one group of body parts per day. You will also be starting to train your heavy sets with more intensity, and you will see an acceleration of the muscular gains. After you have been training for a while, say three to six months, begin to experiment with different training programs, combinations of exercises, and techniques. There are many different valid ways to train, and each has something to offer. An interesting book on sophisticated training approaches is *The Poliquin Principles* by Charles Poliquin. To order it, call 707-257-2348 or go to: http://www.charlespoliquin.net/index.htm.

Another book with an entirely different, more fundamental, approach to training is *Beyond Brawn* by Stuart McRobert, ordered by credit card at http://www.hardgainer.com, or by calling 509-234-0362, or by mailing to CS Publishing, P.O. Box 1002, Connell, WA 99326.

THE 3-DAY SPLIT

On several of these exercises I give you an alternate exercise to use for variety. In the beginning, you should probably stick with one specific exercise for a given body part for a period of four to eight weeks, then use an alternate. Once you become familiar with weight lifting and correct technique, you will want to try some of the other many different variations, and perhaps begin to periodize your training and use more advanced techniques.

Day 1: Chest, Shoulders, Triceps
Barbell flat bench press – 2 w and 1 h set
(Alternate: incline bench press)

Cable side deltoid raise (laterals) – 2 w and 1 h set
Cable rear deltoid raises – 2 w and 1 h set
Triceps pushdowns – 2 w and 1 h set
(Alternate: Close-grip bench press)
Note: Rest one or more days.

Day 2: Back, Biceps, Abdominals
Seated close-grip pulldowns to the stomach – 2 w and 1 h set
Barbell biceps curl – 2 w and 1 h set
(Alternate: preacher bench barbell curls)
Crunches – 3 sets of 10-20 reps
Note: Rest one or more days.

Day 3: Quadriceps, Hamstrings, and Calves (Legs)
Squat – 2 w and 1 h set
(Alternate: Seated leg press)
Again, the squat is the better overall exercise, but some people cannot do it because of back or knee problems.
Lying leg curls – 2 w and 1 h set
Standing calf raises – 2 w and 1 h set
Note: Legs are the most demanding body part, so rest two or more days.

Control the Weight
Studies show that the negative, or return, part of the movement is critical to optimal muscle growth, so do not let the weight fall quickly after lifting it. Exert deliberate control over the negative part of the movement, keeping tension on your muscles through the full range of the movement, and do not rush it.

Making Progress
When you can lift a weight for twelve reps, raise the weight 5 to 10 pounds so that you can only lift about six reps. Then try to increase the number of reps you can lift each time you work out to arrive at twelve reps again, and repeat the progression so that you keep increasing the weight you lift. As you grow

stronger, you will grow bigger muscles. You will probably be pretty sore during your early recovery days. For best recovery and growth let yourself heal so that the soreness goes away, even if this means you leave several days between workouts.

During one high-intensity training period several years ago I learned by studying my workout records that if I wanted to put on weight most quickly, I needed a minimum of eight days of rest before I worked the same body part. This meant that for the type of training I was doing I worked a body part every nine days. If you do not allow enough recovery days between workouts, your progress will be slower. When you log your workouts you can see if you are progressing. If you are not making progress pretty much every workout, try giving yourself another day to recover and see if you do not get stronger at each workout. A very thin, ectomorphic guy I once counseled needed fourteen days between workouts to grow optimally!

Keep in mind that the goal is to gain strength and lean body mass. Usually strength appears to precede size, so you get stronger and then notice that you are getting bigger.

Weight-Lifting Exercises
Flat Bench Barbell Press

This exercise primarily works the pectorals or chest. The anterior deltoids and triceps are also involved. Grip should be a little wider than shoulder width.
Steps:
1. Lie down on your back on a flat bench, with your feet flat on floor.
2. Put your hands on bar slightly wider than your shoulders.
3. Pick up the bar by extending your arms. Lift the weight straight up over your chest for a count of one.
4. Squeeze your chest at the top, hold 1-2 seconds.
5. Slowly lower the bar (over 2 seconds), by allowing

your elbows to flare out away from your body until your upper arm is parallel to the floor. Keep your elbows up toward your shoulders rather than letting them flex down toward your stomach.
6. Repeat.

Alternate: Incline Bench Press

This exercise is basically the same as the flat bench press, but tends to work the upper chest and front of the shoulders a little more.

Cable Side Deltoid Raises (Laterals)

This exercise builds the side deltoid cap, the muscle that gives the wide look – think of cannonball delts. This is not an easy exercise to get at first, but once you learn it you will find it to be a best exercise for shoulders, and it is better than lateral raises with dumbbells.
Steps:
1. With a single handle that is attached to a low cable pulley, and leaning slightly forward (with your left side nearest the cable frame), raise the cable from a position to the side of your stomach up and to the outside of your right shoulder. Do this as if you were swinging a back fist so that you would hit someone behind you with the back of your hand. Be sure to swing the cable in an arc out in front of your body with your arm almost straight, with a slight flex in the elbow rather than letting it stay low as it comes around. Feel yourself resisting the pull of gravity as you move through this arc.
2. The position you end at should be about shoulder height out to your right. Hold this position for 1-2 seconds.
3. Control the negative movement as you let the cable pull your arm in an arc back down to the left side of your stomach to the starting position (over 2 seconds).
4. Repeat.

5. Repeat the entire sequence for the other side, but reverse your position.

Cable Rear Deltoid Raises

This exercise builds your rear deltoid so that you have a deep and wide look. You may see people who seem to have big shoulder caps, but when they turn sideways they disappear. The rear delt completes the shoulders and makes them look much more powerful. Many people miss this.

Steps:

1. With a single handle that is attached to a low cable pulley, and bent over at the waist so that your torso is horizontal, with your left side nearest the cable frame, pull the cable from a position under your body to the left of your left shoulder in an arc up to the outside of your right shoulder. Keep your arm straight or only slightly bent throughout the movement. Avoid flexing your tricep during the movement.
2. Your hand should end at a high position – on the same plane as your head, not down by your stomach. Hold 1-2 seconds.
3. Control the negative movement as you let the cable pull your arm in an arc back down to the side of your left shoulder at the starting position (over 2 seconds).
4. Repeat.
5. Repeat the entire sequence for the other side, but reverse your position.

Triceps Cable Pushdown

This exercise effectively works the triceps as long as you keep the elbows close to the body during the movement. You can do this exercise with a bent bar that has a bend in the middle so that it is shaped like a slight V.

Steps:

1. Stand with your feet hip width apart, bend knees slightly, and put your back to the pad at the overhead pulley machine.

2. Grasp the V-handle bar with overhand grip, palms facing downward.
3. Pull your shoulder blades back, lift chest, and tighten abdominals.
4. By contracting your triceps, straighten your arms, aggressively pushing bar down toward floor.
5. Stop when your arms are fully extended.
6. Squeeze your triceps, hold 1-2 seconds.
7. Without moving upper arms, return to starting position (over 2 seconds).
8. Repeat.

Close-grip Bench Press

This exercise works the triceps with some involvement of the shoulders and chest. Performed somewhat like the standard bench press, only with a closer grip.

Steps:

1. With a grip approximately 14 inches apart, no closer, lower the barbell from over your chest keeping your arms close to your body. The bar should end at a spot just below your pecs, before driving it back up to a lockout position; this keeps the tension on the inner chest and triceps, which is right where you want it.
2. Squeeze your triceps. Hold 1-2 seconds.
3. Return to the starting position (over 2 seconds).
4. Repeat.

Seated Close-grip Overhead Cable Pulldowns

If done properly, this exercise works the entire back (lats).

Steps:

1. Sit on bench with feet flat on floor, abdominals tight.
2. Grasp overhead pulley bar with hands about eight inches apart with palms facing you.
3. From the fully stretched overhead position, pull the bar down to your stomach by bringing your elbows to your sides as you lean back slightly. Be

sure to keep your back arched and firm with your shoulders back.

4. Squeeze your lats in the bottom position. Hold 1-2 seconds.

5. Keeping your back firm, slowly (over 2 seconds) let the bar go up until you are in the fully stretched overhead starting position.

6. Repeat.

Standing Barbell Curls

This exercise works the biceps. The EZ curl bar is best for this but a straight bar can be used.

Steps:

1. Grasp barbell slightly wider than shoulder width, palms facing forward. Pull shoulders back, lift chest. Arms should be fully straightened down at your sides.

2. Stand with feet hip width apart, bend knees slightly, tighten abdominals.

3. By contracting biceps, slowly move barbell in an arc out from the front of the body until the barbell is up to your chest. The hard part is to keep elbows at your sides (stationary) throughout the movement. That is why it is easier to do curls using a bench.

4. Squeeze your biceps at the top, hold 1-2 seconds, keeping your elbows stationary.

5. Slowly return to your starting position (over 2 seconds).

6. Repeat.

Preacher Curl

This exercise works the biceps. Assisting muscles are removed from involvement in this lift, so this isolates the biceps very well. The EZ curl bar is best for this, but a straight bar can be used. Bring the weight all the way to the bottom fully stretched position for full development of the biceps. For any exercise to fully develop a given muscle, it must to through the full range of motion. If you do not go all the way to the bottom, the lower part of the biceps will not grow

as well. Control the weight and do not jerk on the way to the bottom as this can cause injury.

Steps:

1. From the seated position of the preacher bench, grasp the EZ curl barbell at the outside grip position, palms facing forward.

2. By contracting biceps, lift the barbell up to the topmost position.

3. Squeeze your biceps at top and hold 1-2 seconds.

4. Slowly return to the bottom at the starting position (over 2 seconds). Be sure to go all the way down smoothly.

5. Repeat.

Abdominal Crunches on Mat

Primarily works the abdominals.

Steps:

1. Lie flat on your back.

2. Bend knees 90 degrees.

3. Press lower back into floor.

4. Tighten abdominals.

5. Slowly curl your upper body toward your pelvis, leaving your lower back on the mat.

6. When your head is highest off the mat, squeeze your abdominals. Hold 1-2 seconds.

7. Slowly curl your upper body back to the starting position.

8. Repeat.

Note: concentrate on squeezing your abdominals throughout the movement.

Barbell Squats

This most taxing of all exercises primarily works the quadriceps (thigh), but it also involves the gluteals (buttocks), hamstrings and your lower back. This is the exercise that can best re-build a flattened "AZT butt!" It is a difficult exercise that not everyone can perform. Tall lanky people often have trouble doing squats. I recommend the assistance of a competent spotter. Alternative: Smith machine squats.

Steps:

1. Stand up straight with your feet hip width apart. Face straight bar on squat rack.
2. Place the midpoint of the bar across your trapezius muscle (back of neck/shoulder).
3. Place your hands wider than shoulder width to balance the bar, your palms facing forward to grasp the bar.
4. Place your feet hip width apart, facing forward with your knees lined up over your toes.
5. Pull your shoulder blades back, arch your back, chest up, and tighten your abdominals.
6. By bending your knees, smoothly descend to a position where your upper legs are parallel to the floor (about 2 seconds). Be sure to look straight ahead, not down, keep your chest lifted, and maintain a slight arch in your lower back.
7. Contract your quadriceps, and straighten your legs to lift you up to the starting position, as though you are trying to push your feet through the floor (over 1 second).
8. Repeat.

Squats are a difficult exercise to learn to do properly and a short description does not really do it justice. One good book to read to learn to squat properly is *The Insider's Tell-All Handbook on Weight Training Technique*, by Stuart McRobert. You can get it by credit card at www.hardgainer.com or by calling 509-234-0362 or by mailing to CS Publishing, P.O. Box 1002, Connell, WA 99326. Another one is *Super Squats*, by Randall Strossen, Ph.D., ordered by calling 800-447-0008, ext. 1.

Seated Leg Press

This exercise primarily works the quadriceps (or thigh), but it also involves the hamstrings and gluteals. It puts less strain on the back than squats.
Steps:

1. Sit on the machine with your lower back and shoulders against the pad.
2. Place your feet hip width apart on the platform. Contract your quadriceps and straighten your knees to lift the weight to starting position.
3. Pull your shoulders back, tighten your abdominals. Lower the weight by smoothly bending your knees as your legs come down toward your chest (2 seconds).
4. Stop just before your knees touch your chest.
5. Contract your quadriceps and straighten your knees to lift the weight.
6. For maximal effect do not straighten your legs fully, but shop just short of locking the knees and hold for 1-2 seconds. This stresses the quads more.
7. Repeat.

Lying Leg Curl Machine

This exercise works the hamstrings (leg biceps).
Steps:

1. Lie belly down on the leg curl machine, placing the back of your ankles under the pad.
2. Press your abdominals tightly down onto the machine.
3. By contracting hamstrings, slowly bring heels toward buttocks. Stop when you are unable to bring your heels any closer without moving your abdominals. Keep your hips in contact with the machine at all times.
4. Squeeze hamstrings. Hold 1-2 seconds.
5. Slowly return to the starting position (2 seconds).
6. Repeat.

Standing Calf Machine

This exercise works both heads of the calf.
Steps:

1. Stand with your toes on the platform, your heels off the platform, and your knees slightly bent, with the pad on your shoulders.
2. Pull your shoulders back, tighten abdominals.
3. By contracting your calves, rise up on your toes (1 second).

4. Stop when you are as high as you can get on your tiptoes. Squeeze your calves and hold 1-2 seconds.

5. Slowly return to the starting position (2 seconds).

6. Repeat.

Recommended Reading

Below we list some good reading references so that you may gather all the information you need to make informed decisions about the use of our guidelines. We do not agree with everything in these publications, and our concepts may differ considerably with some concepts they contain. However, they all have some merit.

AIDS – Immune System

1. *Healing HIV*, by Jon Kaiser, M.D. Health First Press. Mill Valley, California. Jon's second book shows tremendous evolution in his approach. His wellness-based integrated HIV medical model is designed to build health and strength in the body so that you either do not need to use AIDS drugs or you respond better to lower doses of drugs. Dr. Kaiser believes that you will also have less potential to become resistant to the drugs that are needed. His ideas about addressing hormonal and nutritional deficiencies and improving digestive health should be studied by HIV(+) people and their doctors.

2. *The Guide to Living with HIV Infection*, by John Bartlett, M.D. The Johns Hopkins University Press. 701 West 40th Street, Baltimore, MD, 21211.

3. *How Your Immune System Works*, by Jeff Baggish, M.D. Ziff-Davis Press, 5903 Christie Avenue, Emeryville, CA 94608. This insightful

doctor/author also illustrated this book. It is understandable to everyone.

4. *500 Tips for Coping with Chronic Illness*, by Pamela Jacobs, M.A., Robert Read Publishers, 750 La Playa, Suite 647, San Francisco, CA 94121.

5. *AIDS Treatment News*. The best, single, quick periodical devoted to AIDS research. http://www.aids.org/index.html

6. *Cooking For Life, A Guide To Nutrition and Food Safety for the HIV-Positive Community*, by Robert H. Lehmann. Dell Publishing. Available at most large book stores.

Nutrition

1. *The Real Vitamin & Mineral Book*, by Shari Lieberman, Ph.D. Avery Publishing Group, Garden City Park, New York. This is the best book to give you truly good information on what nutrient doses are effective. Dr. Lieberman understands and recommends the correct higher potencies that have been proven to jobs that lower potencies cannot do.

2. *Mastering The Zone*, by Barry Sears, Ph.D. Harper Collins Publishers, Inc., 10 East 53rd, Street, New York, NY 10022. Learn the principles but avoid the dogma. Numerous people have told us how they have reduced their lipodystrophy symptoms and/or lowered their cholesterol

using the "Zone" approach to eating. To build muscle, eat more calories than he recommends, though.

3. *The Fat Burning Diet*, by Jay Robb. Jay Robb Enterprises, Box 711533, Santee, CA 92072-1533. Call 1 (800) 862-8763 to order. Similar principles as the Zone diet, but not as rigid. Could also be called *Fat-Burning, Muscle Building Diet*, as the information in this book can also apply to building muscle if you get enough calories.

4. *Nutrients as Ergogenic Aids for Sports and Exercise*, by Luke Bucci, Ph.D. CRC Press, Inc. 2000 Corporate Boulevard, N.W., Boca Raton, FL 33431.

5. *Fats that Heal, Fats that Kill*, by Udo Erasmus. Alive Books, 7436 Fraser Park Drive, Burnaby BC, Canada V5J 5B9. This book details how essential fatty acids are critical for optimal health.

6. *Healing Nutrients*, by Patrick Quillin, Ph.D. Random House Publishers, New York, NY.

7. *Flax Oil as a True Aid Against Arthritis, Heart Infarction, Cancer, and Other Diseases*, by Dr. Joanna Budwig. Apple Publishing Company Ltd. 220 East 50th Avenue, Vancouver, British Columbia, Canada V5X 1X9.

8. *Prescription for Nutritional Healing*, by James Balch, M.D. Avery Publishing Group, Inc., Garden City Park, New York.

9. *Nutrition Almanac*, by Lavon J. Dunne. McGraw-Hill Publishing Company, New York, NY.

10. *Sports Supplement Review*, by Bill Phillips. The fact that this book is a very good sales tool for Bill's EAS bodybuilding supplements does not change the fact that he and his staff have produced an insightful guide to bodybuilding supplements that really is the best of its kind. 1 (800) 297-9776.

11. *The Green Pharmacy*, by James Duke, Ph.D. Prevention Books. Available at any book store.

Botanist and former head of the U.S. Department of Agriculture James Duke promotes natural healing with foods and herbs.

12. *Alternative Medicine*. This is one of the best magazines to subscribe to if you are interested in nutrition and alternative or complementary medicine. 1 (360) 385-6021. Like some other alternative medicine groups, they make the mistake of believing that HIV is not involved in causing AIDS, though.

13. *Townsend Letter for Doctors and Patients*. Alternative (nutritional) medicine's oldest journal. 1 (360) 385-6021.

14. *Clinical Pearls News*. CP reviews 5,000 journals and gives a brief synopsis of interesting nutrition studies. Highly recommended. 1 (916) 483-1431.

Anabolic Steroids

1. *Beyond Anabolic Steroids*, by Dr. Mauro Di Pasquale. M.G.D. Press, 23 Main Street, Warkworth, Ontario K0K 3K0. Dr. Di Pasquale is one of the most accurate researchers there is, and each of his books is worthwhile reading.

2. *Anabolic Steroid Side Effects*, by Dr. Mauro Di Pasquale. M.G.D. Press, 23 Main Street, Warkworth, Ontario K0K 3K0.

3. *Anabolic-Androgenic Steroids*, by Charles Kochakian, Ph.D., Springer-Verlag, Berlin, 1976, ISBN 3-540-07710-3. This out-of-print book, edited by the father of anabolic steroids, Dr. Charles Kochakian, starts with the details of Dr. Kochakian's early discoveries in 1935 and provides a solid foundation to understand the metabolism of testosterone and its analogs. Of the numerous academic books on anabolic steroids that could be recommended, including books by Kruskemper, Vida, and others, this is perhaps the best book to read. You will probably only locate it in a university medical library. There are scientific mistakes in it, though. Although it can be hard to locate, this book

continues to be circulated in bodybuilding stores around the world.

4. *Anabolic Reference Guide*, by Bill Philips. Mile High Publishing. P.O. Box 277, Golden, CO 80402. A comprehensive underground guide to the different anabolic steroids. Does not provide medical information, though.

5. *The Underground Steroid Handbook*, by the late Dan Duchaine. This is the most popular underground steroid book of all time because of Dan's irreverence, and the way he tells it like it is. There are scientific mistakes in it, though.

Note: All the currently available underground steroid books contain significant scientific errors. Most of the information they contain is based on anecdotal information rather than medical journal studies, so use them as general guides only.

Weight Training

1. *Beyond Brawn* by Stuart McRobert, ordered at http://www.hardgainer.com, or by calling 1-509-234-0362, or by mailing to CS Publishing, P.O. Box 1002, Connell, WA 99326.

2. *The Poliquin Principles* by Charles Poliquin. Charles Poliquin is an expert physical training coach to elite athletes and Olympic champions. His approach is extremely creative (and humorous). This is a good source of sophisticated weight training techniques. 1 (707) 257-2348. http://www.charlespoliquin.net/index.htm

3. *Heavy-Duty*, by the late Mike Mentzer. Mike's controversial approach can work very well in its context. Is it the only correct method as Mentzer asserted? Michael Mooney trained with Mentzer for ten weeks in 1992 and experienced amazing increases in strength. Elite training coaches like Charles Poliquin and Dragomir Cioroslan credibly contend that building and fine-tuning a physique for strength, aesthetics or competition requires a more varied approach. While we

agree with them, you can learn something valuable from Mentzer's approach – and it is simple. Call 1 (310) 827-7661.

4. *Muscle Meets Magnet*, by Per Tesch, Ph.D. This book uses magnetic resonance imaging (MRI) to show you how certain exercises affect specific muscles. This will help you understand correct training form and how you can target your muscles to shape them for best balance. 1 (800) 447-0008, ext.1.

5. *Ironman's Ultimate Bodybuilding Encyclopedia*, by Peter Sisco. This book has complete details on proper weight-lifting form and technique, and tells you which exercises affect which muscles. 1(800) 447-0008.

6. *Getting Stronger* by Bill Pearl. Great pictures, easy to read. 1(800) 496-8734 or www.amazon.com.

Facial Augmentation and Reconstruction

1. Dewan PA, et al. Histological response to injected Polytef and Bioplastique in a rat model. *Br J Urol* 1994 Apr; 73(4): 370-376.

2. Ersek RA, et al. Bioplastique: a new biphasic polymer for minimally invasive injection implantation. *Aesthetic Plast Surg* 1992 Winter; 16(1): 59-65.

3. Ersek RA, et al. Bioplastique at 6 years: clinical outcome studies. *Plast Reconstr Surg* 1997 Nov; 100(6): 1570-1574.

4. Gold MH. Fibrel. *Dermatol Clin* 1995 Apr; 13(2): 353-361.

5. Jost G. Experience with collagen injection for the correction of contour deficiencies. *Aesthetic Plast Surg* 1985; 9(2): 163-165.

6. Klein AW, et al. Treatment of facial furrows and rhytides. *Dermatol Clin* 1997 Oct; 15(4): 595-607.

7. Lemperle G, et al. PMMA microspheres for intradermal implantation: Part I. Animal research. *Ann Plast Surg* 1991 Jan; 26(1): 57-63.

8. Lemperle G, et al. PMMA-Microspheres (Artecoll) for long-lasting correction of wrinkles correction of wrinkles [see comments]. *Aesthetic Plast Surg* 1998 Sep-Oct; 22(5): 356-365.

9. Mladick RA. Twelve months of experience with Bioplastique. *Aesthetic Plast Surg* 1992 Winter; 16(1): 69-76.

10. Piacquadio D, et al. Evaluation of hylan b gel as a soft-tissue augmentation implant material. *J Am Acad Dermatol* 1997 Apr; 36(4): 544-549.

11. Pieyre JM. Collagen injections: two years' experience. *Aesthetic Plast Surg* 1985; 9(2): 153-154.

12. Simons G, et al. Utilization of injectable microimplants in aesthetic facial surgery. *Aesthetic Plast Surg* 1992 Winter; 16(1): 77-82.

13. West TB, et al. Autologous human collagen and 1dermal fibroblasts for soft tissue augmentation. *Dermatol Surg* 1998 May; 24(5): 510-512.

Personal Testimonials

The first letter is from a man who has experienced the benefits of very progressive use of anabolic steroids. Because everyone is so different, all doctors should be willing to work creatively with a patient to find what gives him or her optimal quality of life. For some people, different dosages will work better. While many men will respond to 100 to 200 mg. per week of testosterone, we have seen others who were highly progressed in AIDS who did not feel normal energy levels until they were given 300 mg. of testosterone along with 300 mg. of nandrolone per week. Quite a difference! With a complex critical illness like HIV/AIDS there is no one-size-fits-all formula.

* * *

Dear Michael:

Back in June I asked you for a reference in New York for a doctor who would prescribe steroids to HIV patients. You sent me to Dr. Doug Dieterich. You also asked that I let you know how I liked him. I must thank you heartfully for the recommendation. Doug sat with me and listened to my story. Mine is not nearly as bad as many. I only lost one lover and one close friend. I myself only had Kaposi's sarcoma, which was "cured" with interferon three years ago. Doug said it sounded like I was depressed. I never thought of it that way. I just thought dragging my butt every day was part of the dark cloud AIDS brought with it.

Doug put me on 200 mg. of testosterone and 2000 mcg. of B12 immediately. I had an energy jump, not to mention the sex drive jump. For the next six weeks I was on 100 mg. of testosterone per week since my testosterone levels seemed to be normal. Still my weight dropped two pounds at this dosage. I had been seeing the nutritionist attached to the clinic. Now I wanted to see the doctor again. I asked for a cycle of Deca and Doug gave me 200 mg. of Deca plus 200 mg. of testosterone immediately. I have not felt this together for 15 years. The drugs have taken away the looming dark cloud and have given me a greater sense of control over my body and consequently helped me to focus my life. Work is better and I have energy to get through the day and still get to the gym. I am more patient with my staff and feel a heightened sense of self-esteem. am very pleased with what has been done at the clinic. I am not certain whether it is the drugs or the plain psychological effect of knowing that I am doing something to help my body beyond just keeping AIDS somewhat capped with protease inhibitors. Thanks so much for the recommendation!

– L. Marks

* * *

Dear Nelson,

If you have not taken time to look around and see the impact your work has had on so many, many lives that would have been lost otherwise . . . please stop and notice. Your work should be getting the same press as the protease inhibitors. I believe it makes that much difference in the quality of life of an HIV-infected person. Thanks for showing me the way to manifest dreams. I love you, Nelson.

– Arlette Pharo, D.O.

* * *

Dear PoWeR,

I have AIDS and had taken on the appearance of a holocaust victim. My lifetime normal weight of 145 lbs. had reached a low of 125 lbs. Six weeks later, following Nelson Vergel's recommended PoWeR program, I weigh more now than I have ever weighed. At 150 lbs. plus, I look and feel great. One fantastic side effect has been the return of a more normal sex life.

– C. Kirby

* * *

Dear PoWeR,

Over a period of approximately 10 months I was facing an ever-increasing list of symptoms including nausea and vomiting, weakness, fatigue, weight loss, and the associated depression. I was just plain sick and felt lousy, but nobody seemed to listen to me. Finally my doctor, Dr. Shannon Schrader, referred me to Nelson Vergel. I spoke with Nelson and he assured me I was a good candidate for his PoWeR program for wellness restoration. He took the time to schedule an appointment in his office in Houston. Nelson was very sympathetic and really understood my frustration and failing health. At last, someone who understood! After only two weeks of following his simple program I gained 10 lbs., and had more energy than I'd had in months. I remember telling Nelson, "my only regret is that I didn't start sooner!" Five weeks have gone by since my initial contact with Nelson, and I have gained 19 lbs. of lean body mass, my energy level has skyrocketed, and I have not even started working out yet. I have not felt this good in many months! As an LVN, I learned much about proper nutrition and exercise, as well as the use of steroids in some HIV wasting cases. Never had it been

explained as thoroughly and simply and applied with such effectiveness, until I had the great fortune to meet Nelson Vergel and begin my own program for wellness restoration. Bravo Nelson! Thank you for giving me hope and showing me that it is possible to feel good again!

– Randy C.

* * *

Dear Michael Mooney,

Thanks so much for your suggestions at the last "Built To Survive" lecture you gave in West Hollywood. I was the one who came up to you with all the joint and tendon problems in knees and elbows from working out. Since your talk I have added acupuncture, Knox Nutri-Joint gelatin (three scoops per day), loose glutamine (two spoonfuls per day), loose glucosamine sulfate (three or four spoons per day) and alpha lipoic acid (800 mg. per day) to the regimen. I have to say that there has been phenomenal improvement in the tendonitis, numbness and ulnar nerve dysfunction in my forearms. I know the alpha lipoic acid works because when I ran out of the pills the pain returned, and it subsided when I started taking them again. I have started working out again for upper body, only two days per week, but the point is that I can work out at all. My knees are still very problematic, but I am confident that this regimen can only increase the chances of their healing more speedily.

With sincere appreciation,
P. Arenson

* * *

Dear Nelson,

I am an HIV-positive . . . hummmm use to think that being positive was a GOOD THING. Well, actually I still do. I have never been so alive since I discovered that I was HIV-positive a couple of years ago – decided to either get crazy and die, or GET REAL and do something fantastic to my body. I was lucky in that the new protease medication was just starting to hit the market. I had a viral load at 14,000 and T4-

cell count of 500. Weight was about 170 lbs., size 33 waist, however, even now without starting on the big O protease yet, I have an undetectable viral load, and T4 count of 800; 172 lbs., size 31 waist (leaner). I am taking Anadrol and working out four days each week. Was taking testosterone cypionate – a 200 mg. injection once per week. My doctor suggested that I try Anadrol to see how it worked with me. I am meeting my doctor today to discuss stacking testosterone cypionate with the Anadrol as I understand that they work better together.

It is a crazy, scary world when you discover that you are HIV-positive. All doctors have different ideas on treatment. Other HIV(+) people have different suggestions for treatment, etc. It is such a wonderful thing to find someone like you folks . . . (Nelson Vergel) . . . that shed light on how we can survive – through such dedication to research done through long, hard hours. THANK YOU, THANK YOU, THANK YOU, THANK YOU.

Your hard work and the lives you save through sharing your knowledge is appreciated by us, and our friends and family that love us and want us around. You are loved.

Thanks (such a simple word for so much),
Jerry

* * *

To Everyone,

After finding myself dying in a hospital at 125 pounds, and then putting on 60 pounds to regain my health, I can say that the information contained in this book is something all HIV(+) people should know about – IT HAS HELPED ME STAY ALIVE. It contains fundamental wellness tools that should be in all our arsenals. Thank you, Michael and Nelson!

– Jeff Taylor, San Diego

* * *

Dear Michael,

I have taken the PoWeR suggestions for eating and steroids quite seriously for the last six months and actually have had my protease pot belly shrink

down so that it's barely sticking out and my triglycerides decrease to the high end of normal. I am currently taking testosterone and Winstrol, and avoiding all sugar and starch, and will continue too, as long as it keeps working. Thank you for giving me your time and your knowledge.

– Mark T.

* * *

Guys,

I've been on a Deca/testosterone regime for about 6 months, and I am very happy with it. I feel like I look like a healthy human again. I have put on about ten pounds of muscle and my face has filled out. My cheeks are still a little drawn, but with the rest of my face filling, you hardly notice it. And my butt has even returned. But most important, the Crix belly has definitely gone down. People have told me I look like I have lost 10 pounds (I've gained it). I know, because my waist size has gone down. Lifting weight with some aerobics is a big part of it, along with the Deca/testosterone I have put on a total of 40 pounds.

– Mark

* * *

Nelson,

Tim here from Dallas. I spoke with you a couple of months ago. Was experiencing dramatic weight loss, dropped to 155 from 175. Started a modified PoWeR cycle. We are now at 200 mg. testosterone and 100 mg. nandrolone every other week. Glad I am almost done since they have stopped manufacturing the generic and the Deca is on back order. The results have been phenomenal, I am now up to 188 lbs. and have gotten noticeably bigger.

Thanks for all the help.
Tim

* * *

BIG THANKS to Michael and Nelson for making me aware of Deca via the PoWeR web site. Last year, when I found out about PoWeR, my doctor (who is fairly progressive) had no knowledge of anabolics and

I had to educate him. I told all of my friends about PoWeR. You guys have helped many people.

Cheers! Jari D.

* * *

In the summer of 1992, I was diagnosed with HIV while pursuing a career as an actor in West Hollywood, California. My dreams seemed to vanish before me as I packed my bags and moved back to my family in Pennsylvania to await death.

Three years later I developed anemia, KS, and lymphoma as my viral load skyrocketed to 750,000 and my T cells fell to 70. Hospitalized for a month I underwent transfusions, chemotherapy and dual antiretroviral therapy. I was told I had 6 months to live. Fortunately, access to the new protease inhibitors brought my viral load down to 1,700 while my T cells rose to 250. Friends from Los Angeles told me of anabolic therapy but my doctor dismissed it as novel and unnecessary.

Determined to survive I gained access to the Internet and surfed to find Medibolics. I hungrily devoured the information and decided to email Michael Mooney. Much to my surprise he emailed me back and a phone conversation soon followed. I found Michael to be the most educated and compassionate man that I have ever spoken to concerning HIV and survival. Once empowered with an arsenal of information I was able to convince my doctor to give me a testosterone test, which showed that I was low at only 200. She put me on the ALZA patch and we both watched as my zest for life and strength increased.

Soon after this we both had the pleasure of attending a lecture in Harrisburg by Nelson Vergel, who shared his personal story and insight. We experimented with Oxandrin, and I gained more weight. Then I saw Dr. Douglas Dieterich of New York, who worked with me using Deca and testosterone with incredible success. Thanks to anabolic therapy I have my life back right where I want it. I am in the best shape of my life, I have become a personal trainer, teach aerobics 6 days per week, and my quality of life is the best ever. This empowerment to survive and the *Built To Survive* handbook have given me the guidelines to a healthy way of life where a person with HIV does not have to look and feel sick. Although I will always have a battle with HIV, I feel that I can meet any challenges that I have to face, and I have much to share to empower others like myself who are facing adversity.

Thank you,
Jim, Harrisburg, PA

* * *

Nelson and Michael,

You are practicing what the scientists only theorize . . . they can learn a lot from your hard work and from the good work of PoWeR.

Thank you,
Ed

* * *

References

[1]Anon. Muscle provides glutamine to the immune system. *Nutri Rev* (1990) 48:390-392.

[2]Ardawi, MS, et al. Metabolism in lymphocytes and its importance in the immune response. *Essays in Biochem* (1985) 21:143.

[3]Newsholme, EA. Psychoimmunology and cellular nutrition: an alternative hypothesis. *Bio Psychiat* (1990) 27:1-3.

[4]Kotler, DP, et al. Magnitude of body-cell-mass depletion and the timing of death from wasting in AIDS. *Am J Clin Nutr* (1989) 50:444-447.

[5]Spaulding, M. Anorexia and appetite stimulation in cancer patients. *Oncol* (1989) 3(suppl):17-23.

[6]Wade, GN, et al. Theoretical review: gonadal effects on food intake and adiposity, a metabolic hypothesis. *Physiol Behav* (1979) 22:583-593.

[7]Hervey, E, et al. Energy storage in female rates with progesterone in absence of increased food intake. *J Physiol* (1967) 200:118-119.

[8]Oster, MH. Megestrol acetate in patients with AIDS. *Ann Int Med* (1994) 15:121(6):400-408.

[9]Harte, C, et al. Progestagens and Cushing's syndrome. *Int J Med Sci* (1995) 165(4):274-275.

[10]Hamburger, AW, et al. Megestrol acetate induced differentiation of 3T3-L1 adipocytes in vitro. *Semin Oncol* (1988) 15(suppl 1):76-78.

[11]Summerbell, DC. Metestrol acetate vs cyproheptadine in the treatment of weight loss associated with HIV infection. *Int J STD AIDS* (1992) 3:278-280.

[12]Furth, PA. Megestrol acetate and cachexia associated with human immunodeficiency virus infection (letter). *Ann Int Med* (1989) 110(8):667.

[13]Henry, K, et al. Diabetes mellitus induced by megestrol acetate in a patient with AIDS and cachexia. *Ann Int Med* (1992) 116(1):53-54.

[14]Von Roenn, JH, et al. Megestrol acetate for treatment of anorexia and cachexia associated with human immunodeficiency virus infection. *Sem Oncol* (1990) 17(suppl 9)(6):13-16.

[15]DiSaia, PJ, et al. Unusual side effect of megestrol acetate. *Am J Obstet Gynecol* (1977) 15(4):460-461.

[16]Kotler, D, et al. Magnitude of body cell mass depletion and timing of death from wasting in AIDS. *Am J Clin Nutr* (1989) 50:444-447.

[17]Muurahainen, N, et al. Detection of occult wasting by BIA technology. Graduate Hospital of Philadelphia. *X International Conference on AIDS, Tokyo* (1994) Aug 7-12; 10(2):220. Abstract No. PB0895.

[18]Sluys, T, et al. Body composition in patients with acquired immunodeficiency syndrome: a validation study of bioelectrical impedance analysis. *J Parent Ent Nutr* (1993) 17(5):404-406.

[19]Wang, J, et al. Body fat measurement in patients with acquired immunodeficiency syndrome: which method should be used? *Am J Clin Nutr* (1992) 56(6):963-967.

[20]Jacobs, DO. Bioelectric impedance analysis: a way to assess changes in body cell mass in patients with AIDS. *J Parent Ent Nutr* (1993) 17(5):401-402.

[21]Denning, DW, et al. Pulmonary Aspergillosis in AIDS. *N Eng J Med* (1991) 324:654-662.

[22]Tindall, B, et al. The Sidney AIDS Project: development of acquired immunodeficiency syndrome in a group of HIV seropositive homosexual men. *Aust N Z J Med* (1988) 18:8-15.

[23]Caiffa, WT, et al. Drug smoking, Pneumocystis carinii pneumonia, and immunosuppression increase risk of bacterial pneumonia in human immunodeficiency virus-seropositive drug users. *Am J Respir Crit Care Med* (1994) 150:1493-1498.

[24]Sherman, MP. Anti-microbial respiratory burst characteristics of pulmonary alveolar macrophages recovered from smokers of marijuana alone, smokers of tobacco alone, smokers of marijuana and tobacco, and nonsmokers. *Am Rev Respir Dis* (1991) 144:1351-1356.

[25]Schwartz, RH, et al. Marijuana to prevent nausea and vomiting in cancer patients: a survey of clinical oncologists. *South Med J* (1997) 90(2):167-172.

[26]Beal, JE, et al. Dronabinol as a treatment for anorexia associated with weight loss in patients with AIDS. *J Pain Sympt Man* (1995) 10:89-97.

[27]Schulte-Beerbuhl, M, et al. Comparison of testosterone, dihydrotestosterone, luteinizing hormone, and follicle-stimulating hormone in serum after injection of testosterone enanthate or testosterone cypionate. *Fert Steril* (1980) 33:201-203.

[28]Nankin, HR. Hormone kinetics after intramuscular testosterone cypionate. *Fertil Steril* (1987) Jun; 47(6):1004-1009.

[29]Vida, JA. *Androgens and Anabolic Agents*, Academic Press: NY/London (1969):16.

[30]Bergink, EW, et al. Metabolism and receptor binding of nandrolone and testosterone under in vitro and in vivo conditions. *Acta Endocrinologica* (1985) 271 (suppl):31-37.

[31]Wijnand, HP, et al. Pharmacokinetic parameters of nandrolone decanoate to healthy volunteers. *Acta Endocrinol Suppl* (Copenh) (1985) 271:19-30.

[32]Welder, AA, et al. Toxic effects of anabolic-androgenic steroids in primary rat hepatic cell cultures. *J Pharmacol Toxicol Methods* (1995) 33(4):187-195.

[33]Marquardt, GH, et al. Failure of non-17-alkylated steroids to produce abnormal liver function tests. *J Clin Endocrinol* (1964) 24:1334-1336.

[34]Gold, J, et al. Safety and efficacy of nandrolone decanoate for treatment of wasting in patients with HIV infection. *AIDS* (1996) 10(7):745-752.

[35]Coodley, GO, et al. A trial of testosterone therapy for HIV-associated weight loss. *AIDS* (1997) 11(11):1347-1352.

[36]Bhasin, S, et al. The effect of supraphysiological doses of testosterone on muscle size and strength in normal men. *N Engl J Med* (1996) Jul 4; 335(1):1-7.

[37]Friedl, KE, et al. Comparison of the effects of high dose testosterone and 19-nortestosterone to a replacement dose of testosterone on strength and body composition in normal men. *J Steroid Biochem Mol Biol* (1991) 40(4-6):607-612.

[38]Kurz, EM, et al. Androgens regulate the dendritic length of mammalian motoneurons in adulthood. *Science* (1986) 232:395-398.

[39]Kantor, MA, et al. Androgens reduce HDL2-cholesterol and increase hepatic triglyceride lipase activity. *Med Sci Sports Exerc* (1985) 17(4):462-465.

[40]Davignon, J, et al. Triglycerides: a risk factor for coronary heart disease. *Atherosclerosis* (1996) 124 (Suppl):S57-64.

[41]Berger, J, et al. Effect of anabolic steroids on HIV-related wasting. *So Med J* (1993) August 86(8):865-866.

[42]Beyler, AL, et al. Reversal by androstanozole of catabolic action of cortisone acetate. *1st International Congress on Endocrinology, Copenhagen Advanced Abstracts of Short Communications* (Fuchs, F. ed) Periodica (1960) p. 829.

[43]Harding, HR, et al. The anti-catabolic activity of anabolic steroids based on the suppression of cortisone acetate (EAc) induction of liver tryptophan pyrrolase. *VI Pan American Congress on Endocrinology, Mexico* (1965).

[44]Salvato, P, et al., *2nd International Conference on Nutrition and HIV Infection, Cannes, France* (1997) April 23-24; Abstract No. 0-003.

[45]Strawford, A, et al. Resistance exercise and supraphysiologic androgen therapy in eugonadal men with HIV-related weight loss: a randomized controlled trial. *JAMA* (1999) Apr 14; 281(14):1282-1290.

[46]Lennon, HD, et al. Anabolic activity of 2-oxa-17alpha-methyldihydrotestosterone (oxandrolone) in castrated rats. *Steroids* (1964) 4:689-697.

[47]Kochakian, CD. Personal communication to Michael Mooney, 1995.

[48]Kotler, DP, et al. Magnitude of body-cell-mass depletion and the timing of death from wasting in AIDS. *Am J Clin Nutr* (1989) 50:444-447.

[49]Schlumpberger, JM, et al. CD8 lymphocyte counts and the risk of death in advanced HIV infection. *J Fam Pract* (1994) 38(1):33-38.

[50]Sattler, FR, et al. Effects of pharmacological doses of nandrolone decanoate and progressive resistance training in immunodeficient patients infected with human immunodeficiency virus. *J Clin Endocrinol Metab* (1999) Apr; 84(4):1268-1276.

[51]Coodley, GO, et al. A trial of testosterone therapy for HIV-associated weight loss. *AIDS* (1997) 11(11):1347-1352.

[52]Rabkin, JG, et al. Testosterone replacement therapy in HIV illness. *Gen Hosp Psychiat* (1995) Jan; 17(1):37-42.

[53]Dobs, AS, et al. Endocrine disorders in men infected with human immunodeficiency virus. *Am J Med* (1988) 84(3, Pt 2):611-616.

[54]Grinspoon, SC, et al. Body composition and endocrine function in women with acquired immunodeficiency syndrome wasting. *J Clin Endocrinol Metab* (1997) 82(5):1332-1337.

[55]Kotler, DP, et al. Magnitude of body-cell-mass depletion and the timing of death from wasting in AIDS. *Am J Clin Nutr* (1989) 50:444-447.

[56]Berger, D, et al. Measurement of Body Weight and Body Cell Mass in Patients receiving Highly Active Antiretroviral Therapy (HAART). *Proceedings ICAAC Conference, Toronto* (1997) October.

[57]Jeantils, V, et al. Weight gain under oral testosterone undecanoate in AIDS. *Therapie* (1993) 48:59-72.

[58]Berger, J, et al. Effect of anabolic steroids on HIV-related wasting myopathy. *So Med J* (1993) August; 86(8):865-866.

[59]Rabkin, JG, et al. Testosterone replacement therapy in HIV illness. *Gen Hosp Psychiatry* (1995) 17(1):37-42.

[60]Gilden, D. Anabolic steroids for wasting. Interview with Dr. Barry Chadsey. *AIDS Treatment News* (1993) #187:4.

[61]Jekot, W, et al. Treating HIV/AIDS patients with anabolic steroids. *AIDS Patient Care* (1993) 3:68-74.

References

[62]Bhasin, S, et al. The effect of supraphysiological doses of testosterone on muscle size and strength in normal men. *N Engl J Med* (1996) 335(1):1-7.

[63]Salvato, P, et al. *2nd International Conference on Nutrition and HIV Infection, Cannes, France* (1997) April 23-24; Abstract No. 0-003.

[64]Strawford, A, et al. Resistance exercise and supraphysiologic androgen therapy in eugonadal men with HIV-related weight loss. *JAMA* (1999) 281(14):1282-1290.

[65]Gold, J, et al. Safety and efficacy of nandrolone decanoate for treatment of wasting in patients with HIV infection. *AIDS* (1996) 10(7):745-752.

[66]Bucher, G, et al. A prospective study on the safety and effect of nandrolone decanoate in HIV-positive patients. *XI International Conference on AIDS, Vancouver* (1996) 11(1):26. Abstract No. Mo.B.423.

[67]Strawford, A, et al. Effects of nandrolone decanoate (ND) on nitrogen balance, metabolism, body composition and function in men with AIDS wasting syndrome (AWS). *2nd International Conference on Nutrition and HIV Infection, Cannes, France* (1997):267.

[68]Hengge, UR, et al. Oxymetholone promotes weight gain in patients with advanced human immunodeficiency virus infection. *Brit J of Nutr* (1996) 75:129-138.

[69]Ott, M, et al. Biolectrical impedance analysis as a predictor of survival in patients with human immunodeficiency virus infection. *J Acquir Immune Def Synd Hum Retro* (1995) 9(1):20-25.

[70]Li, ZG, et al. Effects of gonadal steroids on the production of IL-1 and IL-6 by blood mononuclear cells in vitro. *Clin and Exp Rheum* (1993) 11(2):157-162

[71]Klein, SA, et al. Substitution of testosterone in a HIV positive patient with hypogonadism and wasting syndrome led to a reduced rate of apoptosis. *Eur J Med Res* (1997) 2(1):30-32.

[72]Wagner, G, et al. Illness stage, concurrent medications, and other correlates of low testosterone in men with HIV. *J AIDS Hum Retro* (1995) 8(2):204-207.

[73]Karnieli, E, et al. Insulin resistance in Cushing's syndrome. *Horm Metab Res* (1985) 17(10):518-521.

[74]Oehler, G, et al. Hyperinsulinaemia and impaired glucose tolerance in chronic inflammatory liver disease (author's disease). *Z Gastroenterol* (1981) 19(1):26-32.

[75]Laakso, M. Insulin resistance and coronary heart disease. *Curr Opin Lipidol* (1996) 7(4):217-226.

[76]Björntorp, P. The regulation of adipose tissue distribution in humans. Int J Obes Relat Metab Disord (1996) 20(4):291-302.

[77]Mulligan, KE, et al. Evidence of unique metabolic effects of protease inhibitors. *5th Conf Retrovir Oppor Infect* (1998) Feb 1-5;157 (Abstract No. 414).

[78]Walli, RK, et al. Peripheral insulin resistance leading to impaired glucose tolerance in HIV-1 infected patients treated with protease inhibitors. *Int Conf AIDS, Geneva* (1998)12:777 (Abstract No. 179/41177).

[79]Carr, A, et al. Pathogenesis of HIV-1 protease inhibitor-associated peripheral lipodystrophy, hyperlipidaemia, and insulin resistance. *Lancet* (1998) Jun 20; 351(9119):1881-1883.

[80]Haffner, SM. Decreased testosterone and dehydroepiandrosterone sulfate concentrations are associated with increased insulin and glucose concentrations in nondiabetic men. *Metabol* (1994) 43(5):599-603.

[81]Haffner, SM. Decreased testosterone and dehydroepiandrosterone sulfate concentrations are associated with increased insulin and glucose concentrations in nondiabetic men. *Metabol* (1994) 43(5):599-603.

[82]Armellini, F, et al. Interrelationships between intraabdominal fat and total serum testosterone levels in obese women. *Metabolism* (1994) 43(3):390-5.

[83]Engelson, ES, et al. Nutrition and testosterone status in HIV-positive women. *XI International Conference on AIDS, Vancouver* (1996) Abstract Tu. B.2382.

[84]Benbrik, E, et al. Cellular and mitochondrial toxicity of zidovudine (AZT) didanosine (ddI) and zalcitabine (ddC) on cultured human muscle cells. *J Neurol Sci* (1997) 149(1):19-25.

[85]Kotler, DP, et al. Magnitude of body-cell-mass depletion and the timing of death from wasting in AIDS. *Am J Clin Nutr* (1989) 50:444-447.

[86]Greene, JB, et al. Clinical approach to weight loss in the patient with HIV infections. *Gastro Clinics of No Amer* (1988) 17(3):573-576.

[87]Hellerstein, MK, et al. Increased de novo hepatic lipogenesis in human immunodeficiency virus infection. *J Clin Endocrinol Metab* (1993) 76(3):559-565.

[88]Laudat, A, et al. Changes in systemic gonadal and adrenal steroids in asymptomatic human immunodeficiency virus-infected men: relationship with the CD4 cell counts. *Eur J Endocrinol* (1995) 133(4):418-424.

[89]Grinspoon, SC, et al. Loss of lean body and muscle mass correlates with androgen levels in hypogonadal men with acquired immunodeficiency syndrome and wasting. *J Clin Endocrinol Metab* (1996) 81(11):4051-4058.

[90]Grinspoon, SC, et al. Body composition and endocrine function in women with acquired immunodeficiency syndrome wasting. *J Clin Endocrinol Metab* (1997) 82(5):1332-1337.

[91]Parsch, CJ, et al. Injectable testosterone undecanoate has more favourable pharmacokinetics and pharmacodynamics than testosterone enanthate. *Euro J of Endo* (1995) 132:514-519.

[92]Rabkin, JG, et al. Testosterone replacement therapy for HIV-infected men. *The AIDS Reader* (1995) July/August:136-144.

[93]Martin, ME, et al. Alterations in the concentrations and binding properties of sex steroid binding protein and corticosteroid-binding globulin in HIV-positive patients. *J Endocrinol Invest* (1992) 15(8):597-603.

[94]Marin, P, et al. Androgen replacement of middle aged, obese men: effects on metabolism, muscle, and adipose tissues. *Eur J Med* (1992) 1(6):329-336.

[95]Moller, J. *Cholesterol: Interactions with Testosterone and Cortisol in Cardiovascular Disease*, Springer-Verlag: Berlin (1987).

[96]Friedl, KE, et al. The administration of pharmacological doses of testosterone or 19-nortestosterone to normal men is not associated with increased insulin secretion or impaired glucose tolerance. *J Clin Endocrinol Metab* (1989) May 68(5):971-5.

[97]Hobbs, CJ, et al. Nandrolone, a 19-nortestosterone, enhances insulin-independent glucose uptake in normal men. [see comments] *J Clin Endocrinol Metab* (1996) 81(4):1582-1585.

[98]Woodard, TL, et al. Glucose intolerance and insulin resistance in aplastic anemia treated with oxymetholone. *J Clin Endocrinol Metab* (1981) 53(5):905-908.

[99]Kailin, X, et al. Hyperinsulinemia accompanying hyperglycemia in Chinese patients with aplastic anemia. *Am J Hematol* (1997) 56(3):151-4.

[100]Kantor, MA, et al. Androgens reduce HDL2-cholesterol and increase hepatic triglyceride lipase activity. *Med Sci Sports Exerc* (1985) 17(4):462-5.

[101]Applebaum-Bowden D, et al. The dyslipoproteinemia of anabolic steroid therapy: increase in hepatic triglyceride lipase precedes the decrease in high-density lipoprotein 2 cholesterol. *Metab* (1987) 36(10):949-952.

[102]Dieterich, D, et al. Incidence of body habitus changes in a cohort of 700 HIV-infected patients. *Infect Diseases Soc Amer* (1998) Nov 12 - 15. Abstract No. 477.

[103]Torres, RA, et al. Treatment of dorsocervical fat pads (buffalo hump) and truncal obesity with Serostim (recombinant human growth hormone) in patients with AIDS maintained on HAART. *XII International AIDS Conference, Geneva* (1998) June 28-July 3. Abstract No. 32164.

[104]Henricksson, J, et al. Influence of exercise on insulin sensitivity. *J Cardio Risk* (1995) 2(4):303-309.

[105]McCarty, MF, et al. Reduction of free fatty acids may ameliorate risk factors associated with abdominal obesity. *Med Hypotheses* (1995) 44(4):278-286.

[106]Truswell, AS. Food carbohydrates and plasma lipids – an update. *Am J Clin Nutr* (1994) 59(suppl)(3):S710S-S718.

[107]Miller, JC, et al. Replacing starch with sucrose in a high glycaemic index breakfast cereal lowers glycaemic and insulin responses. *Eur J Clin Nutr* (1994) 48(10):749-752.

[108]Pamies-Andreu, E, et al. High-fructose feeding elicits insulin resistance without hypertension in normal mongrel dogs. *Am J Hypertens* (1995) 8(7):732-738.

[109]Chen, YD, et al. Why do low-fat high-carbohydrate diets accentuate postprandial lipemia in patients with NIDDM? *Diabetes Care* (1995) 18(1):10-16.

[110]Sheard, NF. The diabetic diet: evidence for a new approach. *Nutr Rev* (1995) 53(1):16-18.

[111]Garg, A, et al. Effects of varying carbohydrate content of diet in patients with non-insulin-dependent diabetes mellitus [see comments]. *JAMA* (1994) 271(18):1421-1428.

[112]Storlien, LH, et al. Influence of dietary fat composition on development of insulin resistance in rats. Relationship to muscle triglyceride and omega-3 fatty acids in muscle phospholipid. *Diabetes* (1991) 40(2):280-289.

[113]Berry, EM. Dietary fatty acids in the management of diabetes mellitus. *Am J Clin Nutr* (1997) 66(4 Suppl):991S-997S.

[114]Yam, D, et al. Diet and disease – the Israeli paradox: possible dangers of a high omega-6 polyunsaturated fatty acid diet. *Isr J Med Sci* (1996) 32(11):1134-1143.

[115]Liu, S, et al. Dietary omega-3 and polyunsaturated fatty acids modify fatty acid composition and insulin binding in skeletal-muscle sarcolemma. *Biochem J* (1994) 299 (Pt 3):831-837.

[116]Ponte, E, et al. Cardiovascular disease and omega-3 fatty acids. *Minerva Med* (1997) 88(9):343-53.

[117]Mori, TA, et al. Interactions between dietary fat, fish, and fish oils and their effects on platelet function in men at risk of cardiovascular disease. *Arterioscler Thromb Vasc Biol* (1997) 17(2):279-286.

[118]Tatsuhiro, M, et al. Beef tallow diet decreases lipoprotein lipase activities in brown adipose tissue, heart, and soleus muscle in reducing sympathetic activities in rats. *J Nutr Sci Vitaminol* (1994) 40:569-581

[119]Okuno M, et al. Perilla oil prevents the excessive growth of visceral adipose tissue in rats by down-regulating adipocyte differentiation. *J Nutr* (1997) 127(9):1752-1757.

[120]Ascherio, A, et al. Health effects of trans fatty acids. *Am J Clin Nutr* (1997) 66(4 Suppl):1006S-1010S.

[121]Lemon, PW, et al. Do athletes need more dietary protein and amino acids? *Int J Sports Nutri* (1995) 5:S39-S61.

[122]Lemon, PW, et al. Protein requirements and muscle mass strength changes during intensive training in novice bodybuilders. *J Appl Physiol* (1992) 73(2):767-775.

References

[123]Boirie, Y, et al. Slow and fast dietary proteins differently modulate postprandial protein accretion. *Proceedings of the National Academy of Science USA* (1997) 94: 14930-14935.

[124]Wilson, BE, et al. Effects of chromium supplementation on fasting insulin levels and lipid parameters in healthy, non-obese young subjects. *Diabetes Res Clin Pract* (1995) 28(3):179-184.

[125]Anderson, RA, et al. Elevated intake of supplemental chromium improves glucose and insulin variables in individuals with type 2 diabetes. *Diabetes* (1997) 46:1786-1791.

[126]Velussi, M, et al. Long-term (12 months) treatment with an antioxidant drug (silymarin) is effective on hyperinsulinemia, exogenous insulin need and malondialdehyde levels in cirrhotic diabetic patients. *J of Hepatol* (1997) 26:871-879.

[127]Jacobs, S, et al. Enhancement of glucose disposal in patients with type 2 diabetes by alpha-lipoic acid. *Drug Res* (1995) 45:872-874.

[128]Estrada, EH, et al. Stimulation of glucose uptake by the natural coenzyme a-lipoic acid/thioctic acid. *Diabetes* (1996) 45:1798-1804.

[129]Busse, E, et al. Influence of alpha-lipoic acid on intracellular glutathione in vitro and in vivo. *Arzneimittel-Forshung* (1992) 42:829-831.

[130]Herzenberg L, et al. Glutathione deficiency is associated with impaired survival in HIV disease. *Proceedings of the National Academy of Sciences USA* (1997) 94(5):1967-1972.

[131]De Simone, C, et al. High dose L-carnitine improves immunologic and metabolic parameters in AIDS patients. *Immunopharmacol Immunotoxicol* (1993) 15(1):1-12.

[132]Hellerstein, MK, et al. Effects of dietary n-3 fatty acid supplementation in men with weight loss associated with the acquired immune deficiency syndrome: Relation to indices of cytokine production. *J AIDS Hum Retro* (1996)11(3):258-270.

[133]Faure, P, et al. Vitamin E improves the free radical defense system potential and insulin sensitivity of rats fed high fructose diets. *J Nutr* (1997) 127(1):103-107.

[134]Basualdo, CG, et al. Vitamin A (retinol) status of first nation adults with non-insulin-dependent diabetes mellitus. *J Am Coll Nutr* (1997) 16(1):39-45.

[135]Mak, RH, et al. The vitamin D/parathyroid hormone axis in the pathogenesis of hypertension and insulin resistance in uremia. *Miner Electrolyte Metab* (1992) 18(2-5):156-159.

[136]Sanchez, M, et al. Oral calcium supplementation reduces intraplatelet free calcium concentration and insulin resistance in essential hypertensive patients. *Hypertension* (1997) 29(1 Pt 2):531-536.

[137]Facchini, F, et al. Relation between dietary vitamin intake and resistance to insulin-mediated glucose disposal in healthy volunteers. *Am J Clin Nutr* (1996) 63(6):946-949.

[138]Nadler, JL, et al. Magnesium deficiency produces insulin resistance and increased thromboxane synthesis. *Hypertension* (1993) 21(6 Pt 2):1024-1029.

[139]Baum, M, et al. Inadequate dietary intake and altered nutrition status in early HIV-1 infection. *Nutrition* (1994) 10(1):16-20.

[140]Baum, MK, et al. Micronutrients and HIV-1 disease progression. *AIDS* (1995) 9(9):1051-1056.

[141]Reddi, A, et al. Biotin supplementation improves glucose and insulin tolerances in genetically diabetic KK mice. *Life Sci* (1988) 42(13):1323-1330.

[142]Koutsikos, D, et al. Oral glucose tolerance test after high-dose i.v. biotin administration in normoglucemic hemodialysis patients. *Ren Fail* (1996) 18(1):131-137.

[143]Koutsikos D, et al. Biotin for diabetic peripheral neuropathy. *Biomed Pharmacother* (1990) 44(10):511-514.

[144]Devara, JS, et al. The effects of alpha tocopherol supplementation on monocyte function. Decreased lipid oxidation interleukin 1 beta secretion and monocyte adhesion to endothelium. *J Clin Invest* (1996) 98(3):756-763.

[145]Munoz, JA, et al. Effect of vitamin C on lipoproteins in healthy adults. *Ann Med Interne* (Paris) (1994) 145(1):13-19.

[146]Peterson, JC, et al. Vitamins and progression of atherosclerosis in hyperhomocysteinemia. *Lancet* (1998) Jan 24, 351(9098):263.

[147]Refsum, H, et al. Homocysteine and cardiovascular disease. *Annu Rev Med* (1998) 49:31-62.

[148]Hickson, RC, et al. Glutamine prevents down regulation of myosin heavy chain synthesis and muscle atrophy from glucocorticoids. *Am J Physiol [Endo Metab]* (1995) 269(31):E730-E734.

[149]Hong, RW, et al. Glutamine preserves liver glutathione after lethal hepatic injury. *Ann Surg* (1992) 215(2):114-119.

[150]Opara, EC, et al. L-glutamine supplementation of a high fat diet reduces body weight and attenuates hyperglycemia and hyperinsulinemia in C57BL/6J mice. *J Nutr* (1996) 126(1):273-279.

[151]Borel, MJ, et al. Parenteral glutamine infusion alters insulin-mediated glucose metabolism. *J Parenter Enteral Nutr* (1998) 22(5):280-285.

[152]Guthrie, R. Treatment of non-insulin-dependent diabetes mellitus with metformin. *J Am Board Fam Pract* (1997) 10(3):213-221.

[153]O'Neal, DN, et al. The effect of 3 months of recombinant human growth hormone (GH) therapy on insulin and glucose-mediated glucose disposal and insulin secretion in GH-deficient adults: a minimal model analysis. *J Clin Endocrinol Metab* (1994) 79(4):975-983.

[154]Móldrup, A, et al. Multiple growth hormone-binding proteins are expressed on insulin-producing cells. *Mol Endocrinol* (1989) 3(8):1173-1182.

[155]Gelato, MC, et al. Improved Insulin Sensitivity and Body Fat Distribution in HIV-Infected Patients Treated With Rosiglitazone: A Pilot Study. *JAIDS* (2002); 31(2):163-170.

[156]Thompson, PD, et al. Contrasting effects of testosterone and stanozolol on serum lipoprotein levels. *J Am Med Assoc* (1989) 261(8):1165-1168.

[157]Glazer, G., et al. Lack of demonstrated effect of nandrolone on serum lipids. *Metabolism* (1994) 43(2):204-210.

[158]Hara, T, et al. Oxandrolone and plasma triglyceride reduction: effect on triglyceride-rich and high-density lipoproteins. *Artery* (1981) 9(5):328-341.

[159]Reeves, RD, et al. Hyperlipidemia due to oxymetholone therapy. Occurrence in a long-term hemodialysis patient. *J Am Med Assoc* (1976) 236(5):469-472.

[160]Zgliczynski, S, et al. Effect of testosterone replacement therapy on lipids and lipoproteins in hypogonadal and elderly men. *Atherosclerosis* (1996) 121(1):35-43.

[161]Hanash, KA, et al. Androgen effect on prostate specific antigen secretion. *J Surg Oncol* (1992) 49(3):202-204.

[162]Svetec, DA, et al. The effect of parenteral testosterone replacement on prostate specific antigen in hypogonadal men with erectile dysfunction. *J Urol* (1997) 158(5):1775-1777.

[163]Douglas, TH, et al. Effect of exogenous testosterone replacement on prostate-specific antigen and prostate-specific membrane antigen levels in hypogonadal men. *J Surg Oncol* (1995) 59(4):246-250.

[164]Gann, PH, et al. Prospective study of sex-hormone levels and risk of prostate cancer. *J Natl Cancer Inst* (1996) 88(16):1118-1126.

[165]Ribeiro, M, et al. Low serum testosterone and a younger age predict for a poor outcome in metastatic prostate cancer. *Am J Clin Oncol* (1997) 20(6):605-608.

[166]Monda, LM, et al. The correlation between serum prostate-specific antigen and prostate cancer is not influenced by the serum testosterone concentration. *Urology* (1995) 46(1):62-64.

[167]Suzuki, K, et al. Endocrine environment of benign prostatic hyperplasia: prostate size and volume are correlated with serum estrogen concentration. *Scand J Urol Nephrol* (1995) 29:65-68.

[168]Gann, PH, et al. A prospective study of plasma hormone levels, nonhormonal factors, and development of benign prostatic hyperplasia. *The Prostate* (1995) 26:40-49.

[169]Marquardt, GH, et al. Failure of non-17-alkylated steroids to produce abnormal liver function tests. *J Clin Endocrinol* (1964) 24:1334-1336.

[170]Welder, AA, et al. Toxic effects of anabolic-androgenic steroids in primary rat hepatic cell cultures. *J Pharmacol Toxicol Methods* (1995) 33(4):187-195.

[171]Hickson, RC, et al., Adverse effects of anabolic steroids. *Med Toxicol Adv Drug Exp* (1989) 4:254-271.

[172]Ishak, KG, et al. Hepatotoxic effects of the anabolic/androgenic steroids. *Semin Liver Dis* (1987) 7(3):230-236.

[173]Kosaka, A, et al. Hepatocellular carcinoma associated with anabolic steroid therapy: report of a case and review of the Japanese literature. *J Gastroenterol* (1996) 31(3):450-454.

[174]Hernandez-Nieto, L, et al. Benign liver-cell adenoma associated with long-term administration of an androgenic-anabolic steroid (methandienone). *Cancer* (1977) 40(4):1761-1764.

[175]Rabkin, JG, et al. Testosterone treatment of clinical hypogonadism in patients with HIV/AIDS. *Int J STD AIDS* (1997) 8:537-545.

[176]Metzger, DL, et al. Estrogen receptor blockade with tamoxifen diminishes growth hormone secretion in boys: evidence for a stimulatory role of endogenous estrogens during male adolescence. *J Clin Endocrinol Metab* (1994) 79(2):513-518.

[177]el-Sheikh, MM, et al. The effect of Permixon (saw palmetto) on androgen receptors. *J Acta Obstet Gynecol Scand* (1988) 67(5):397-399.

[178]Suzuki, K, et al. Endocrine environment of benign prostatic hyperplasia: prostate size and volume are correlated with serum estrogen concentration. *Scand J Urol Nephrol* (1995) 29:65-68.

[179]Gann, PH, et al. A prospective study of plasma hormone levels, nonhormonal factors, and development of benign prostatic hyperplasia. *The Prostate* (1995) 26:40-49.

[180]Trattner, A, et al. The appearance of Kaposi's sarcoma during corticosteroid therapy. *Cancer* (1993) Sep. 1; 72(5):1779-1783.

[181]Guo, W, et al. Increased levels of glucocorticoid receptors (GR) expression in AIDS-Kaposi's sarcoma. Meeting Abstract. *Proceedings of the Annual Meeting of the American Association of Cancer Research* (1993) 34:A3016

[182]Schulhafer, EP, et al. Steroid-induced Kaposi's sarcoma in a patient with pre-AIDS. *Am J Med* (1987) Feb:82(2): 313-317.

[183]Martin, RW, et al. Kaposi's Sarcoma. *Medicine* (1993)72:245-261.

[184]Rosenthal, E, et al. Estrogen, progesterone, and androgen and their receptors in epidemic Kaposi's sarcoma. *IX International Conference on AIDS, Berlin* (1993) Jun 6-11; 9(1):403. Abstract No. PO-B12-1605.

[185]Christeff, N, et al. Differences in androgens of HIV positive with and without KS. *East Parisian CISIH Group. International Conference on AIDS, Berlin* (1993) Jun 6-11; 9(1):400. Abstract No. PO-B12-1588.

[186]Klauke, S, et al. Sex hormone as a cofactor in the pathogenesis of the epidemic of Kaposi's sarcoma. *AIDS* (1995) 9(11):1295-1296.

[187]Shoefer, H, et al. Kaposi's sarcoma (HIV-positive and HIV) in caucasian women. *International Conference on AIDS, Berlin* (1993) Jun 6-11; 9(1):397. Abstract No. PO-B12-1569.

[188]Lunardi, IY, et al. Tumorigenesis and metastasis of neoplastic KS cell lines in immunodeficient mice blocked by a human pregnancy hormone. *Nature* (1995) May 4; 375(652):64-68.

References

[189]*Positively Aware*, July/August,1995:8.

[190]Ooshika, N, et al. Effect of an anabolic steroid on cellular immunity and postoperative evaluation of uterine cervical cancer. *Jap J of Canc Chemo* (1984) 11(10):2177-2184.

[191]Mendenhall, CL, et al. Anabolic steroid effects on immune function: differences between analogues. *J Ster Biochem Molec Biol* (1990) 37(1):71-76.

[192]Calabrese, LH, et al. The effect of anabolic steroids and strength training on the human immune system. *Med Sci Sports Exerc* (1989) 21(4):386-392.

[193]Huys, JV, et al. Effect of nandrolone decanoate on T-Cell lymphocytes during radiotherapy. *Clin Therap* (1979) 2(5):352-357.

[194]Bucher, G, et al. A prospective study on the safety and effect of nandrolone decanoate in HIV-positive patients. *XI International Conference on AIDS, Vancouver* (1996) 11(1):26. Abstract No. Mo.B.423.

[195]Ansar, AS, et al. Sex hormones, immune responses, and autoimmune diseases. Mechanisms of sex hormone action. *Am J Pathol* (1985) 121(3):531-551.

[196]Marquardt, GH, et al. Failure of non-17-alkylated steroids to produce abnormal liver function tests. *J Clin Endocrinol* (1964) 24:1334-1336.

[197]Welder, AA, et al. Toxic effects of anabolic-androgenic steroids in primary rat hepatic cell cultures. *J Pharmacol Toxicol Meth* (1995) 33(4):187-195.

[198]Haupt, HA, et al. Anabolic steroids: a review of the literature. *Am J Sports Med* (1984) 12(6):469- 484.

[199]Dickerman, RD, et al. Anabolic steroid-induced hepatotoxicity: is it overstated? *Clin J Sport Med* (1999) 9(1):34-39.

[200]Kotler, DP, et al. Magnitude of body-cell-mass depletion and the timing of death from wasting in AIDS. *Am J Clin Nutr* (1989) 50:444-447.

[201]Ehriches, L. Testosterone may prevent AIDS wasting. *Fam Pract* (1994) Oct. 10:36.

[202]Jekot, WF, et al. Treating HIV/AIDS patients with anabolic steroids. *AIDS Patient Care* (1993) April; 7(2):11-17.

[203]Gilden, D. Weight loss: a role for growth hormone and anabolic steroids. *AIDS Treatment News* (1993) Nov 19; 187:16.

[204]Ooshika, N, et al. Effect of an anabolic steroid on cellular immunity and postoperative evaluation of uterine cervical cancer. *Jap J of Canc Chemo* (1984) 11(10):2177-2184.

[205]Calabrese, LH, et al. The effect of anabolic steroids and strength training on the human immune system. *Med Sci Sports Exerc* (1989) Aug; 21(4):386-392.

[206]Huys, JV, et al. Effect of nandrolone decanoate on T-cell lymphocytes during radiotherapy. *Clin Ther* (1979) 2(5):352-357.

[207]Plum, J. Influence of nandrolone decanoate on the repopulation of the thymus after total body irradiation of mice. *Immunopharm* (1982) 5:19.

[208]Ansar, AS, et al. Sex hormones, immune responses, and autoimmune diseases. Mechanisms of sex hormone action. *Am J Pathol* (1985) Dec; 121(3):531-551.

[209]Ahmed, SA, et al. Sex hormones and the immune system. *Ballieres Clinic Rheumat* (1990) Apr; 4(1):13-31.

[210]Gilden, D. Weight loss: a role for growth hormone and anabolic steroids. *AIDS Treatment News* (1993) Nov 19; 187:16.

[211]Dobs, AS, et al. Endocrine disorders in men infected with human immune-deficiency virus. *Am J Med* (1988) 84(3, pt 2):611-661.

[212]Grinspoon, SÇ, et al. Body composition and endocrine function in women with acquired immunodeficiency syndrome wasting. *J Clin Endocrinol Metab* (1997) 82(5):1332-1337.

[213]Hunt, CD, et al. Effects of dietary zinc depletion on seminal volume and zinc loss, serum testosterone concentrations, and sperm morphology in young men. *Am J Clin Nutr* (1992) Jul; 56(1):148-157.

[214]Akaza, N, et al. Effects of vitamin A deficiency on the function of the pituitary-gonadal system in male rats. *Nippon Juigaku Zasshi* (1989) Dec; 51(6):1209-1217.

[215]Sanchez-Capelo, A, et al. Potassium regulates plasma testosterone and renal ornithine decarboxylase in mice. *FEBS Lett* (1993) Oct. 25; 333(1-2):32-34.

[216]Dobs, AS, et al. Serum hormones in men with human immunodeficiency virus-associated wasting. *J Clin Endocrinol Metab* (1996) 81(11):4108-4112.

[217]Klein, SA, et al. Substitution of testosterone in an HIV-1 positive patient with hypogonadism and wasting-syndrome led to a reduced rate of apoptosis. *Eur J Med Res* (1997) 2(1):30-32.

[218]Laudat, A, et al. Changes in systemic gonadal and adrenal steroids in asymptomatic human immunodeficiency virus-infected men: relationship with the CD4 T-cell counts. *Eur J Endocrinol* (1995) 133(4):418-424.

[219]Wagner, GJ, et al. A comparative analysis of standard and alternative antidepressants in the treatment of human immunodeficiency virus. *Compr Psychiatry* (1996) 37(6):402-408.

[220]Simpkins, JW, et al. Variable effects of testosterone on dopamine activity in several microdissected regions in the preoptic area and medial basal hypothalamus. *Endocrinol* (1983) 112(2):665-669.

[221]Sherwin, BB, et al. Androgen enhances sexual motivation in females: a prospective, crossover study of sex steroid administration in the surgical menopause. *Psychosom Med* (1985) 47(4):339-351.

[222]Kaplan, HS, et al. The female androgen deficiency syndrome. *J Sex Marital Ther* (1993) 19(1):3-24.

[223]Svetec, DA, et al. The effect of parenteral testosterone replacement on prostate specific antigen in hypogonadal men with erectile dysfunction. *J Urol* (1997) 158(5):1775-1777.

[224]Douglas, TH, et al. Effect of exogenous testosterone replacement on prostate-specific antigen and prostate-specific membrane antigen levels in hypogonadal men. *J Surg Oncol* (1995) 59(4):246-250.

[225]Suzuki, K, et al. Endocrine environment of benign prostatic hyperplasia: prostate size and volume are correlated with serum estrogen concentration. *Scand J Urol Nephrol* (1995) 29:65-68.

[226]Gann, PH, et al. A prospective study of plasma hormone levels, nonhormonal factors, and development of benign prostatic hyperplasia. *The Prostate* (1995) 26:40-49.

[227]Severson, K, et al. Free testosterone as a predictor for body composition changes in males with HIV or AIDS. *XI International Conference on AIDS, Vancouver* (1996) 11(1):332. Abstract No. Tu.B.2385.

[228]Grinspoon, SÇ, et al. Loss of lean body and muscle mass correlates with androgen levels in hypogonadal men with acquired immunodeficiency syndrome and wasting. *J Clin Endocrinol Metab* (1996) 81(11):4051-4058.

[229]Strain, G, et al. The relationship between serum levels of insulin and sex hormone-binding globulin in men: the effect of weight loss. *J Clin Endocrinol Metab* (1994) 79(4):1173-1176.

[230]Dickerman, RD, et al. Anabolic steroid-induced hepatotoxicity: is it overstated? *Clin J Sport Med* (1999) 9(1):34-39.

[231]Ahmed, SR, et al. Transdermal testosterone therapy in the treatment of male hypogonadism. *J Clin Endocrinol Metab* (1988) 66(3):546-551.

[232]Coodley, GO, et al. A trial of testosterone therapy for HIV-associated weight loss. *AIDS* (1997) 11(11):1347-1352.

[233]Friedl, KE, et al. Comparison of the effects of high dose testosterone and 19-nortestosterone to a replacement dose of testosterone on strength and body composition in normal men. *J Steroid Biochem Mol Biol* (1991) 40(4-6):607-612.

[234]Wagner, GJ, et al. Testosterone therapy for clinical symptoms of hypogonadism in eugonadal men with AIDS. *Int J STD & AIDS* (1998) 9:a1119.1-a1119.4

[235]Kruskemper, HL. Anabolic Steroids. *Academic Press* (NY/London) (1968):59.

[236]Lemon, PW, et al. Do athletes need more dietary protein and amino acids? *Int J Sports Nutri* (1995) 5:S39-S61.

[237]Lemon, PW, et al. Protein requirements and muscle mass/strength changes during intensive training in novice bodybuilders. *J Appl Physiol* (1992) 73(2):767-775.

[238]Bhasin, S, et al. The effect of supraphysiological doses of testosterone on muscle size and strength in normal men. *N Engl J Med* (1996) Jul 4; 335(1):1-7.

[239]Harman, M, et al. Reproductive hormones in aging men. Measurement of sex steroids, luteinizing hormone, and leydig cell response to human chorionic gonadotropin. *J Clin Endocrinol Metab* (1980) 51(1):3540.

[240]Ronnberg, L, et al. Clomiphene citrate administration to normogonadotropic subfertile men: blood hormone changes and activation of acid phosphatase in seminal fluid. *Int J Androl* (1981) 4:372-378.

[241]Lunardi-Iskandar, Y, et al. Tumorigenesis and metastasis of neoplastic Kaposi's sarcoma cell line in immunodeficient mice blocked by a human pregnancy hormone. *Nature* (1995) 375(6526):64-68.

[242]Sanford, LM. Evidence that estrogen regulation of testosterone secretion in adult rams is mediated by both indirect (gonadrotropin dependent) and direct (gonadotropin independent) means. *J Androl* (1985) 6:306-314.

[243]Burge, MR, et al. Idiopathic hypogonadotropic hypogonadism in a male runner is reversed by clomiphene citrate. *Fertil Steril* (1997) 67(4):783-785.

[244]Horikawa, R, et al. Growth hormone and insulin-like growth factor I stimulate Leydig cell steroidogenesis. *Eur J Pharmacol* (1989) 166(1):87-94.

[245]Morales, AJ, et al. The effect of six months treatment with a 100 mg daily dose of dehydroepiandrosterone (DHEA) on circulating sex steroids, body composition and muscle strength in age-advanced men and women. *Clin Endocrinol* (Oxf) (1998) 49(4):421-432.

[246]Clark, RA, et al. Clinical manifestations and predictors of survival in older women infected with HIV. *J AIDS Hum Retro* (1997) 15(5):341-345.

[247]*National Institute of Health News Release*. NJLBI Stops Trial of Estrogen Plus Progestin Due to Increased Breast Cancer Risk, Lack of Overall Benefit. 2002 Jul 9:1-4.

[248]Fletcher SW, et al. Failure of Estrogen Plus Progestin Therapy for Prevention. *JAMA* 2002 Jul 17;288(3):366-368.

[249]Writing Group for the Women's Health Initiative Investigators. Risks and Benefits of Estrogen Plus Progestin in Healthy Postmenopausal Women. *JAMA* (2002) Jul 17; 288(3):321-333.

[250]Yarasheski, KE, et al. Effect of growth hormone and resistance exercise on muscle growth in young men. *Am J Physiol* (1992) 262 (Endocrinol Metab 25): E261-E267.

[251]Yarasheski, KE, et al. Effect of resistance exercise and growth hormone on bone density in older men. *Clin Endocrinol* (Oxf) (1997) 47(2):223-229.

References

[252]Yarasheski, KE, et al. Growth hormone effects on metabolism, body composition, muscle mass, and strength. *Exerc Sport Sci Rev* (1994) 22():285-312.

[253]Bigland, B, et al. Muscle performance in rats, normal and treated with growth hormone. *J. Physiol* 116:129-136,1952.

[254]Yarasheski, KE, et al. Weight-lifting exercise is more effective than rhGH administration for increasing muscle strength in HIV-infected individuals. *Abstract #437.1, FASEB J.* 14(4):A571, 2000.

[255]Salvato, P, et al. *Conference on Nutrition and HIV Infection Cannes, France* (1997) April 23-24; Abstract No. 0-003

[256]Berger, JR, et al. Effect of anabolic steroids on HIV-related wasting myopathy. *So Med J* (1993) Aug; 86(8):865-866.

[257]Berger, JR, et al. Oxandrolone in AIDS-wasting myopathy. *AIDS* (1996) Dec; 10:1657-1662.

[258]Fu, YK, et al. Growth hormone augments superoxide anion secretion of human neutrophils by binding to the prolactin receptor. *J Clin Invest* (1992) 89(2):451-457.

[259]Smith, JA. Neutrophils, host defense, and inflammation: a double-edged sword. *J Leukoc Biol* (1994) 56(6):672-686.

[260]Weissmann, G, et al. Neutrophils: release of mediators of inflammation with special reference to rheumatoid arthritis. *Ann N Y Acad Sci* (1982) 389:11-24.

[261]Zachwieja, JJ, et al. Growth hormone administration in older adults: effects on albumin synthesis. *Am J Physiol* (1994) 266(6 Pt 1):E840-844.

[262]Yarasheski, KE, et al. Effect of growth hormone and resistance exercise on muscle growth and strength in older men. *Am J Physiol* (1995) 268(2 Pt 1):E268-276.

[263]Zachwieja, JJ, et al. Does growth hormone therapy in conjunction with resistance exercise increase muscle force production and muscle mass in men and women aged 60 years or older? *Phys Ther* (1999) 79(1):76-82.

[264]Mulligan, K, et al. Anabolic effects of recombinant human growth hormone in patients with wasting associated with human immunodeficiency virus infection. *J Clin Endocrinol Metab* (1993) 77(4):956-962.

[265]Mulligan, K, et al. Anabolic effects of recombinant human growth hormone in patients with wasting associated with human immunodeficiency virus infection. *J Clin Endocrinol Metab* (1993) 77(4):956-962.

[266]Solerte, SB, et al. Hormonal and chronobiological impairment of GH-IGF1-IGFBP3 axis in HIV infected patients (CDC C3) with wasting syndrome. Effects of treatment with recombinant human GH. *XI International AIDS Conference*, Vancouver (1996) Abstract No. Mo. B.420.

[267]Stoll, BA. Breast cancer risk in Japanese women with special reference to the growth hormone-insulin-like growth factor axis. *Jpn J Clin Oncol* (1992) Feb; 22(1):1-5.

[268]Westley, BR, et al. Role of insulin-like growth factors in steroid modulated proliferation. *J Ster Biochem Mol Biol* (1994) Oct; 51(1-2):1-9.

[269]Malozowski, S. et al. Prepubertal gynecomastia during growth hormone therapy. *J Pediatr* (1995) 126(4):659-661.

[270]Cohn, L, et al. Carpal tunnel syndrome and gynaecomastia during growth hormone treatment of elderly men with low circulating IGF-I concentrations. *Clin Endocrinol* (Oxf) (1993) 39(4):417-425.

[271]Fuh, G, et al. Prolactin receptor antagonists that inhibit the growth of breast cancer cell lines. *J Biol Chem* (1995) 270(22):1313-1317.

[272]Strawford, A, et al. Effects of nandrolone decanoate (ND) on nitrogen balance, metabolism, body composition and function in men with AIDS wasting syndrome (AWS). *2nd International Conference on Nutrition and HIV Infection, Cannes, France* (1997):267.

[273]Björntorp, P. The regulation of adipose tissue distribution in humans. *Int J Obes Relat Metab Disord* (1996) 20(4):291-302.

[274]Jeevanandam, M, et al. Altered lipid kinetics in adjuvant recombinant human growth hormone-treated multiple-trauma patients. *Am J Physiol* (1994) 267(4, Pt 1):E560-E565.

[275]Hellerstein, MK, et al. Increased de novo hepatic lipogenesis in human immunodeficiency virus infection. *J Clin Endocrinol Metab* (1993) 76(3):559-565.

[276]Rodgers, BD, et al. Catabolic hormones and growth hormone resistance in acquired immunodeficiency syndrome and other catabolic states. *Proceedings of the Society of Experimental Biology and Medicine* (1996) Sep; 212(4):324-331.

[277]Solerte, SB, et al. Hormonal and chronobiological impairment of GH-IGF1-IGFBP3 axis in HIV infected patients (CDC C3) with wasting syndrome. Effects of treatment with recombinant human GH. *XI International AIDS Conference, Vancouver* (1996) Abstract No. Mo. B.420.

[278]G'omez de Segura, IA, et al. Comparative effects of growth hormone in large and small bowel resection in the rat. *J Surg Res* (1996) 62(1):5-10.

[279]Berni Canani, R, et al. Comparative effects of growth hormone on water and ion transport in rat jejunum, ileum, and colon. *Dig Dis Sci* (1996) 41(6):1076-1081.

[280]Allen, RE, et al. Regulation of skeletal muscle satellite cell proliferation and differentiation by transforming growth factor-beta, insulin-like growth factor I, and fibroblast growth factor. *J Cell Physiol* (1989) 138(2):311-315.

[281]Rudman D, et al. Effects of human growth hormone in men over 60 years old [see comments]. *N Engl J Med* (1990) 323(1):1-6 1990.

[282]Lashner, BA, et al. The effect of folic acid supplementation on the risk of cancer or dysplasia in ulcerative colitis. *Gastroenterol* (1997) 112:29-32.

[283]Knox KK, et al. Active infection by variant A of human herpes virus six causes destruction of lymphoid tissues of HIV infected individuals. *40th ICAAC*, Sept. 17-20, 2000 Toronto, Ontario, Canada; Abstract #787.

[284]Miller, JC, et al. Replacing starch with sucrose in a high glycaemic index breakfast cereal lowers glycaemic and insulin responses. *Eur J Clin Nutr* (1994) 48(10):749-752.

[285]Hadjivassiliou, M, et al. Does cryptic gluten sensitivity play a part in neurological illness? *Lancet* (1996) 347(8998):369-371.

[286]Volek, JS, et al. Testosterone and cortisol in relationship to dietary nutrients and resistance exercise. *J Appl Physiol* (1997) 82(1):49-54.

[287]Kremer, JM, et al. Dietary fish oil and olive oil supplementation in patients with rheumatoid arthritis. Clinical and immunologic effects. *Arthritis Rheum* (1990) 33(6):810-820.

[288]Biolo, G, et al. An abundant supply of amino acids enhances the metabolic effect of exercise on muscle protein. *Am J Phys* (1997) 36:E122-E129.

[289]Okamura, K, et al. Effect of amino acid and glucose administration during post exercise recovery on protein kinetics in dogs. *Am J Physiol* (1997) 272(6, Pt 1): E1023-E1030.

[290]Boirie, Y, et al. Slow and fast dietary proteins differently modulate postprandial protein accretion. *Proceedings of the National Academy of Sciences USA* (1997) 94:14930-14935.

[291]Mocchegiani, E, et al. Benefit of oral zinc supplementation as an adjunct to zidovudine (AZT) therapy against opportunistic infections in AIDS. *Int J Immunopharmacol* (1995) 17(9):719-727.

[292]Bounous, G, et al. Whey protein as a food supplement in HIV-seropositive individuals. *Clin & Invest Med* (1993) Jun; 16(3): 204-209.

[293]Bounous, G, et al. Immunoenhancing property of dietary whey protein in mice: role of glutathione. *Clin & Invest Med* (1989) 12:154-161.

[294]Bounous, G, et al. The biological activity of undenatured dietary whey proteins: the role of glutathione. *Clin & Invest Med* (1991) 14(4):296-309.

[295]Bogstedt, AK, et al. Passive immunity against diarrhea. *Acta Paediatr* (1996) Feb; 85(2):125-128.

[296]Liani, RM, et al. Lactoferrin inhibits HIV-1 replication in vitro and exhibits synergy when combined with zidovudine. *AIDS* (1999) Jul 9;13(1):1273-1274.

[297]Berkhout, B, et al. Characterization of the anti-HIV effects of native lactoferrin and other milk proteins and protein-derived peptides. *Antiviral Res* (2002) Aug;55(2):341-355. bberkhout@amc.uva.nl.

[298]Munster, AM, et al. The effect of antibiotics on cell-mediated immunity. *Surgery* (1977) 81(6): 692-695.

[299]Hubbard, L, et al. *Lifeline*; Loma Linda University (1990) 5:6.

[300]Floyd, JC, et al. Stimulation of insulin secretion by amino acids. *J Clin Invest* (1966) Sep 45:1487.

[301]Eaton, SB, et al. Paleolithic nutrition. A consideration of its nature and current implications. *N Eng J Med* (1985) 312(5): 283-289.

[302]Freed, DJ, et al. Anabolic steroids in athletics: crossover double-blind trial on weightlifters. *Br Med J* (1975) 2(59):471-473.

[303]Hum, S. Varied protein intake alters glutathione metabolism in rats. *J Nutri* (1992) 122(10):2010-2018.

[304]Lemon, PW, et al. Do athletes need more dietary protein and amino acids? *Int J Sports Nutri* (1995) 5:S39-S61.

[305]Baum, M, et al. Inadequate dietary intake and altered nutrition status in early HIV-1 infection. *Nutrition* (1994) 10(1):16-20.

[306]Bogden, JD, et al. Daily micronutrient supplements enhance delayed-hypersensitivity skin test responses in older people. *Am J Clin Nutr* (1994) 60(3):437-447.

[307]Chandra, RK, et al. Effect of vitamin and trace-element supplementation on immune responses and infection in elderly subjects. *Lancet* (1992) 340 (8828):1124-1127.

[308]Abrams, B, et al. A prospective study of dietary intake and AIDS in HIV-positive homosexual men. *J AIDS* (1993) 6:949-958.

[309]Franken, DG, et al. Treatment of mild hyperhomocysteinemia in vascular disease patients. *Arterioscler Thromb* (1994) 14(3):465-470.

[310]Ubbink, JB, et al. The effect of a subnormal vitamin B-6 status on homocysteine metabolism. *J Clin Invest* (1996) 98(1):177-184.

[311]Mantero-Atienza, E, et al. Vitamin B6 and immune function in HIV infection. *VI International Conference on AIDS* (1990) 6(2):432 Abstract No. 3123.

[312]Shor-Posner, G, et al. Anxiety and depression in early HIV-1 infection and its association with vitamin B6 status. *VIII International Conference on AIDS* (1992) 8(2):B209. Abstract No. POB 3711.

[313]Tang, AM, et al. The effect of micronutrient intake on survival in HIV-1 infection. *XI International Conference on AIDS, Vancouver* (1994) 10(2):220. Abstract No. PB0894.

[314]Tang, AM, et al. Low serum vitamin B-12 concentrations are associated with faster human immunodeficiency virus type 1 (HIV-1) disease progression. *J Nutr* (1997) 127(2):345-351.

[315]Baum, MK, et al. Micronutrients and HIV-1 disease progression. *AIDS* (1995) 9(9):1051-1056.

[316]Beach, RS, et al. Plasma vitamin B12 level as a potential cofactor in studies of human immunodeficiency virus type 1-related cognitive changes. *Arch Neurol* (1992) 49(5):501-506.

[317]den Heijer, M, et al. Vitamin supplementation reduces blood homocysteine levels: a controlled trial in patients with venous thrombosis and healthy volunteers. *Arterioscler Thromb Vasc Biol* (1998) 18(3):356-361.

References

[318]Gallagher, PM, et al. Homocysteine and risk of premature coronary heart disease. Evidence for a common gene mutation. *Circulation* (1996) 94(9):2154-2158.

[319]Young, SN, et al. Folic acid and psychopathology. *Prog Neuropsychopharmacol Biol Psychiatry* (1989) 13(6):841-863.

[320]*Harper's Biochemistry*, 24th Ed. Appleton & Lange, Stamford, Conn. Page 614.

[321]Brubacher GB, et al. The vitamin A activity of beta-carotene. *Int J Vitam Nutr Res* 985;55(1):5-15.

[322]Basualdo, CG, et al. Vitamin A (retinol) status of first nation adults with non-insulin-dependent diabetes mellitus. *J Am Coll Nutr* (1997) (1):39-45.

[323]Akaza, N, et al. Effects of vitamin A deficiency on the function of the pituitary-gonadal system in male rats. *Nippon Juigaku Zasshi* (1989) Dec; 51(6):1209-1217.

[324]Evain-Brion, D, et al. Vitamin A deficiency and nocturnal growth hormone secretion in short children. *The Lancet* (1994) 343:87-88.

[325]Greenberg, BL, et al. Vitamin A deficiency and maternal-infant transmissions of HIV in two metropolitan areas in the United States. *AIDS* (1997) 11(3):325-332.

[326]Semba, RD, et al. Increased mortality associated with vitamin A deficiency during human immunodeficiency virus type 1 infection. *Arch Intern Med* (1993) 153(18):2149-2154.

[327]Sibulesky L, et al. Safety of <7500 RE (<25000 IU) vitamin A daily in adults with retinitis pigmentosa. *Am J Clin Nutr* (1999) Apr; 69(4):656-663.

[328]Pastorino U, et al. Safety of high-dose vitamin A. Randomized trial on lung cancer chemoprevention. *Oncology* (1991);48(2):131-117.

[329]Neuhouser ML, et al. Absorption of dietary and supplemental folate in women with prior pregnancies with neural tube defects. *J Am Coll Nutr* (1998) Dec; 17(6):625-630.

[330]Johnston, CS. Biomarkers for establishing a tolerable upper intake level for vitamin C. *Nutr Rev* (1999) Mar; 57(3):71-77.

[331]Meydani, SN, et al. Vitamin E supplementation and in vivo immune response in healthy elderly subjects. A randomized controlled trial. *J Am Med Assoc* (1997) 277:1380-1386.

[332]Devaraj, S, et al. The effects of alpha tocopherol supplementation on monocyte function: decreased lipid oxidation, interleukin 1 beta secretion, and monocyte adhesion to endothelium. *J Clin Invest* (1996) 98(3):756-763.

[333]Faure, P, et al. Vitamin E improves the free radical defense system potential and insulin sensitivity of rats fed high fructose diets. *J Nutr* (1997) 127(1):103-107.

[334]Tang, AM, et al. Association between serum vitamin A and E levels and HIV-1 disease progression. *AIDS* (1997) 11(5):613-620.

[335]Allard, JP, et al. Effects of vitamin E and C supplementation on oxidative stress and viral load in HIV-infected subjects. *AIDS* (1998) 12(13):1653-1659.

[336]Sanchez, M. et al. Oral calcium supplementation reduces intraplatelet free calcium concentration and insulin resistance in essential hypertensive patients. *Hypertension* (1997) 29(1 Pt 2):531-536.

[337]Perez-Rodriguez, E, et al. The role of calcium supplements in the treatment of nelfinavir-induced diarrhea. *39th ICAAC, Sept. 26-29, 1999 San Francisco, California. Abstract #1308.*

[338]Tang, AM, et al. Effects of micronutrient intake on survival in human immunodeficiency virus type 1 infection. *Am J Epidem* (1996) 143(12):1244.

[339]Koch, J, et al. Zinc levels and infections in hospitalized patients with AIDS. *Nutrition* (1996) 12(7-8):515-518.

[340]Hunt, CD, et al. Effects of dietary zinc depletion on seminal volume and zinc loss, serum testosterone concentrations, and sperm morphology in young men. *Am J Clin Nutr* (1992) Jul; 56(1):148-157.

[341]Dorup, A, et al. Role of insulin-like growth factor-1 and growth hormone in growth inhibition induced by magnesium and zinc deficiencies. *Br J Nutr* (1991) Nov; 66(3):505-521.

[342]Arens M, et al. Zinc salts inactivate clinical isolates of herpes simplex virus in vitro. *J Clin Microbial* (2000) May; 38(5):1758-1762.

[343]Petrus E, et al. Randomized, double-matched, placebo-controlled, clinical study of the effectiveness of zinc acetate lozenges on common cold symptoms in allergy-tested subjects. *Cur Thera Res* (1998) September; 59:595-607.

[344]Dworkin, BM, et al. Abnormalities of blood selenium and glutathione peroxidase activity in patients with acquired immunodeficiency syndrome and AIDS-related complex. *Biol Trace Elem Res* (1988) 15:167-177.

[345]Baum, MK, et al. Risk of HIV-related mortality is associated with selenium deficiency. *J AIDS Hum Retro* (1997) 15:370-376.

[346]Anderson, RA, et al. Elevated intake of supplemental chromium improve glucose and insulin variables in individuals with type 2 diabetes. *Diabetes* (1997) 46:1786-1791.

[347]Boelaert, JR, et al. Altered iron metabolism in HIV infection: mechanisms, possible consequences, and proposals for management. *Inf Agents & Dis* (1996) 5(1):36-46.

[348]Dandona, P, et al. Insulin resistance and iron overload. *Ann Clin Biochem* (1983) 20 Pt 2:77-79.

[349]Gordeuk, VR, et al. Carbonyl iron therapy for iron deficiency anemia. *Blood* (1986) Mar; 67(3):745-52.

[350]Omara, FO, et al. Vitamin E is protective against iron toxicity and iron-induced hepatic vitamin E depletion in mice. *J Nutrition* (1993) Oct; 123(10):1649-1655.

351Sprince, H, et al. Protective action of ascorbic acid and sulfur compounds against acetaldehyde toxicity: implications in alcoholism and smoking. *Agents Actions* (1975) 5(2):164-273.

352Sprince, H, et al. Protection against acetaldehyde toxicity in the rat by L-cysteine, thiamin and L-2-methylthiazolidine-4-carboxylic acid. *Agents Actions* (1974) 4(2):125-130.

353Estrela, JM, et al. The effect of cysteine and N-acetyl cysteine on rat liver glutathione (GSH). *Biochem Pharmacol* (1983) 32(22):3483-3485.

354Herzenberg, L, et al. Glutathione deficiency is associated with impaired survival in HIV disease. *Proceedings of the National Academy of Sciences USA* (1997) 94(5):1967-1972.

355De Flora, S, et al. Attenuation of influenza-like symptomology and improvement of cell-mediated immunity with long-term N-acetylcysteine treatment. *Euro Respir Journal* (1997) 10:1535-1541.

356Busse, E, et al. Influence of alpha-lipoic acid on intracellular glutathione in vitro and in vivo. *Arzneimittel-Forshung* (1992) 42:829-831.

357Packer, L, et al. Neuroprotection by the metabolic antioxidant a-lipoic acid. *Free Rad Biol & Med* (1997) 22(1/2):359-378.

358De Simone, C, et al. High dose L-carnitine improves immunologic and metabolic parameters in AIDS patients. *Immunopharmacol Immunotoxicol* (1993) 15(1):1-12.

359Famularo, G, et al. Acetyl-carnitine deficiency in AIDS patients with neurotoxicity on treatment with antiretroviral nucleoside analogues. *AIDS* (1997) 11(2):185-190.

360Lowitt, S, et al. Acetyl-L-carnitine corrects the altered peripheral nerve function of experimental diabetes. *Metabolism* (1995) 44(5):677-680.

361Rai, G, et al. Double-blind, placebo controlled study of acetyl-l-carnitine in patients with Alzheimer's dementia. *Curr Med Res Opin* (1990) 11(10):638-647.

362Moretti, S, et al. Effect of L-carnitine on human immunodeficiency virus-1 infection-associated apoptosis: a pilot study. *Blood* (1998) 91(10):3817-3824.

363Oda, T, et al. Effect of lactobacillus acidophilus on iron bioavailability in rats. *J Nutr Sci Vitaminol* (Tokyo) (1994) 40(6):613-616.

364Ferenci, P, et al. Randomized controlled trial of silymarin treatment in patients with cirrhosis of the liver. *J Hepatol* (1989) 9:105-113.

365Hikino, H, et al. *Planta Medica* (1984) 50: 248-250.

366Wagner, H. Plant constituents with anti-hepatotoxic activity. In: Beal, J., & Reinhard, E., eds. Natural Products as Medicinal Agents (Stuttgart, Germany). *Hippokrates-Verlag* (1981) pp. 545-558.

367Hickson, RC, et al. Glutamine prevents downregulation of myosin heavy chain synthesis and muscle atrophy from glucocorticoids. *Am J Physiol* (1995) 268 (4, Pt 1): E730-E734.

368Hankard, RG, et al. Effect of glutamine on leucine metabolism in humans. *Am J Physiol* (1996) 271(4, pt 1):E748-E754.

369Li, J, et al. Effect of glutamine-enriched total parenteral nutrition on small intestinal gut-associated lymphoid tissue and upper respiratory tract immunity. *Surgery* (1997) 121(5):542-549.

370Ardawi, MS, et al. Glutamine metabolism in lymphocytes and its importance in the immune response. *Essays in Biochemistry* (1985).

371Anon. Muscle provides glutamine to the immune system. *Nutr Rev* (1990) 48:390-392.

372Hong, RW, et al. Glutamine preserves liver glutathione after lethal hepatic injury. *Ann Surg* (1992) 215(2):114-119.

373Skubitz, KM, et al. Oral glutamine to prevent chemotherapy-induced stomatitis: a pilot study. *J Lab Clin Med* (1996) 127(2):223-228.

374Prang, E, et al. L-glutamine promotes gain in weight and body cell mass in patients with AIDS. *International Conference on AIDS Wasting* (1997).

375Souba, WW, et al. Anabolic steroids support postoperative gut/liver amino acid metabolism. *J Parent Ent Nutr* (1988) 12(6):550-554.

376Nestler, JE, et al. Dehydroepiandrosterone reduces serum low density lipoprotein levels and body fat but does not alter insulin sensitivity in normal men. *J Clin Endocrinol Metab* (1988) 66(1):57-61.

377Morales, AJ, et al. Effects of replacement dose of dehydroepiandrosterone in men and women of advancing age. *J Clin Endocrinol Metab* (1994) 78(6):1360-1367.

378Wolkowitz, OM, et al. Dehydroepiandrosterone (DHEA) treatment of depression. *Biol Psych* (1997) 41:311-318.

379Schwartz, AG, et al. Cancer prevention with dehydroepiandrosterone and non-androgenic structural analogs. *J Cell Biochem Suppl* (1995) 22:210-217.

380Henderson, E, et al. Dehydroepiandrosterone (DHEA) and synthetic DHEA analogs are modest inhibitors of HIV-1 IIIB replication. *AIDS Res Hum Retroviruses* (1992) 8(5):625-631.

381Danenberg, HD, et al. Dehydroepiandrosterone protects mice from endotoxin toxicity and reduces tumor necrosis factor production. *Antimicrob Agents Chemother* (1992) 36(10):2275-2279.

382Yang, JY, et al. Inhibition of 3'azido-3'deoxythymidine-resistant HIV-1 infection by dehydroepiandrosterone in vitro. *Biochem Biophys Res Commun* (1994) Jun 30; 201(3):1424-1432.

383Jacobson, MA, et al. Decreased serum dehydroepiandrosterone is associated with an increased progression of human immunodeficiency virus infection in men with CD4 cell counts of 200-499. *J Infect Dis* (1991) 164(5):864-868.

384Jones, JA, et al. Use of DHEA in a patient with advanced prostate cancer: a case report and review. *Urology* (1997) 50(5):784-788.

References

[385]Laudat, A, et al. Changes in systemic gonadal and adrenal steroids in asymptomatic human immunodeficiency virus-infected men:relationship with the CD4 T-cell counts. *Eur J Endocrinol* (1995) 133(4):418-424.

[386]Simpkins, JW, et al. Variable effects of testosterone on dopamine activity in several microdissected regions in the preoptic area and medial basal hypothalamus. *Endocrinol* (1983) 112(2):665-669.

[387]Wehling, M. Looking beyond the dogma of genomic steroid action: insights and facts of the 1990's. *J Mol Med* (1995) 73(9):439-447.

[388]Wolf, RF, et al. Growth hormone and insulin reverse net whole body and skeletal muscle protein catabolism in cancer patients. *Ann Surg* (1992) 216(3):280-290.

[389]Ritchie, WP, Jr. Other causes of GI musosal injury: upper intestinal content. *Clin Invest Med* (1987) 10(3):264-269.

[390]Bolin, T, et al. Decreased lysophospholipase and increased phospholipase A2 activity in ileal mucosa from patients with Crohn's disease. *Digestion* (1984) 29(1):55-59.

[391]Weisser, B, et al. Oxidized low-density lipoproteins in atherogenesis: possible mechanisms of action. *J Cardiovasc Pharmacol* (1992) 19 (suppl 2):S4-S7.

[392]Buyukgebiz, A, et al. Treatment of constitutional delay of growth and puberty with oxandrolone compared with growth hormone. *Arch Dis Child* (1990) 65(4):448-449.

[393]Howard, CP, et al. Children with growth hormone deficiency: intermittent treatment with somatropin and oxandrolone. *Am J Dis Child* (1981) 135(4):326-328.

[394]Rosenfeld, RG, et al. Growth hormone therapy of Turner's syndrome: beneficial effect on adult height. *J Pediatr* (1998) 132(2):319-324.

[395]Nilsson, KO, et al. Improved final height in girls with Turner's syndrome treated with growth hormone and oxandrolone. *J Clin Endocrinol Metab* (1996) 81(2):635-640.

[396]Zambelli, et al. Effect of two different diets on AIDS patients' nutritional status. *Xl International AIDS Conference Vancouver* (1996) Abstract Th.B.4243.

[397]Boirie, Y, et al. Slow and fast dietary proteins differently modulate postprandial protein accretion. *Proceedings of the National Academy of Science USA* (1997) 94: 14930-14935.

[398]Bounous, G, et al. Immunoenhancing property of dietary whey protein in mice: role of glutathione. *Clin & Invest Med* (1989) 12:154-161.

[399]Bounous, G, et al. The biological activity of undenatured dietary whey proteins: the role of glutathione. *Clin & Invest Med* (1991) 14(4):296-309.

[400]Bogstedt, AK, et al. Passive immunity against diarrhoea. *Acta Paediatr* (1996) 85(2):125-128.

[401]Olson, PE, et al. CD4 correlates of weight-training in HIV-seropositive outpatients. *2nd Nat. Conf on Human Retroviruses and Related Infections Washington, D.C.* (1995) Jan. 29-Feb 2. Abstract 544.

[402]Spence, DW, et al. Progressive resistance exercise: effect on muscle function and anthropometry of a select AIDS population. *Arch Phys Med Rehabil* (1990) 71(9):644-648.

[403]Rigsby, LW, et al. Effects of exercise training on men seropositive for the human immunodeficiency virus-1. *Med Sci Sports Exerc* (1992) 24(1):6-12.

[404]Bolinder, J, et al. Site differences in insulin receptor binding and insulin action in subcutaneous fat of obese females. *J Clin Endocr Metab* (1983) 57:455-461.

[405]Bruning, PF, et al. Insulin resistance and breast-cancer risk. *Int J Cancer* (1992)52(4):511-516.

[406]Singh, PN, et al. Dietary risk factors for color cancer in a low-risk population. *Am J Epidemiol* (1998) 148(8):761-774.

[407]Gerber, M. Energy balance and cancers. *Eur J Cancer Prev* (1999) 8(2):77-89.

Index

Index

CMV, 3, 41, 131

coenzyme Q10, 54, 55, 124, 129

colitis, 15, 105, 136

College Pharmacy, 84

Conant, Dr. Marcus, 74

Coodley, 25, 85

copper, 127, 128

corticoid steroids, 15

cortisol, 17, 22, 82, 92

creatine, 36, 88, 119, 136-137

creatine monohydrate, 136

Crix belly, 42, 186

Crixivan, 21, 42, 44, 81, 121, 137

Cryptosporidia, 144

Cushing's syndrome, 42

cytomegalovirus, 131

D

Deca Durabolin, 2, 25, 30, 38, 45-46, 75, 87, 133, 148

Deeks, Dr., 35

dehydroepiandrosterone, 133

delta-9-tetrahydracannabinol, 21

DHEA, 22, 73, 80, 82, 94, 133-134

diabetes, 17, 50, 53, 111, 113, 129, 142; and insulin resistance, 42, 43, 44, 46, 47

diarrhea, 2, 7, 27, 41, 48, 50, 82, 107, 118, 141; and GH, 103; and sucralose use, 113-114; and higher fat diet, 115; and caseine use, 117; and Ritonavir, 122; and Vitamin C, 126; and calcium, 127; and acidophilus, 130-131; and L-Glutamine, 132-133, 137; and ImmunePro, 140; and protease inhibitors, 144-147

Deterich, Dr. Douglas, 46, 163, 166

Digestive Aids, 130

Digestive Enzymes, 147

dihydroanandrolone, 24

dihydrotestosterone, 22, 24, 27, 85

Dobs, Dr. Adrian, 32

dronabinol, 21

Dube, Dr. Michael, 51

Dullnig, Michael, MD, 3, 4, 30

E

edema, 100

electrolyte supplements, 147

EPA, 49, 124, 129, 130

essential fatty acid, 54, 130

estradiol, 73, 82, 94

evening primrose oil, 72, 129

exercise, 2, 4, 6-9, 21, 37, 112, 119, 148-161; and BIA, 19; and testosterone, 37; aerobic-type, 46-47; during steroid cycling, 87; and anabolic agents, 97; and hyperplasia, 102; and orthomolecular nutrition, 137; for children, 140

F

facial wasting, 58, 62-63; *also see:* wasting

finesteride, 68

flax oil, 130, 161

folic acid, 50, 55, 105, 122, 125

Fortovase/Saquinavir, 115

free testosterone, 23, 44, 73, 80, 82, 86, 94, 137, 149

G

Gallo, Dr. Robert, 73

GGT, 76, 83

GH, 13-14, 38-41, 46, 70, 71, 81, 82, 94-102, 139

Giardia, 142, 144

Gill, Dr. Prakesh, 74

GLA, 129, 130

glutamic acid, 130-131

glutamine (L-glutamine), 11-12, 41, 50, 129, 137, 139, 140, 147, 165; and the liver, 29, 72; source of, 48; and

diarrhea, 50; and caseine, 117; in dietary plan, 124; as an important amino acid, 131-133; glutamyl-cysteine, 117-118

glutathione, 29, 49, 78, 120, 127, 129, 133, 140; and N-acetyl-cysteine, 56; and Immunocal, 117-118

glycemic indexes, 47

Glycyrrhizinate Forte, 72

Gold, Dr. Julian, 25, 30, 38, 97

Gorbach, Dr. Sherwood, 44

Great Smokies, 9, 82, 108, 145

Greiff, Dr. Barry, 10

Grinspoon, Dr. Steven, 32

growth hormone (GH), 28, 71, 94, 96, 100-102, 126, 147; the Serostim Human, 38-39, 46, 50

Grunfeld, Dr. Carl, 28, 29

gynecomastia, 22, 24, 28-29, 71, 78, 87, 101

H

hair loss, 24, 68, 77, 78, 87, 90, 93, 135; and testosterone use, 22, 25-26, 68, 77; and stanozolol, 36; in women, 45; and Testoderm, 85

HCG, 41, 69, 70, 73-74, 92-94, 149

HDL, 26, 65

Healing HIV [Kaiser, Dr. Jon], 9, 104, 159

Hellerstein, Dr. Marc, 20, 38, 102

hematocrit, 23, 28, 30, 70, 72, 81, 83, 137

hemoglobin, 23, 72, 81, 130, 137

hepatitis, 42, 66, 72, 75, 76, 83, 142

homocysteine, 50, 125

hormone replacement therapy (HRT), 94-95

Houston Buyers Club, 5, 7, 138, 152

human growth hormone, 13, 38, 46, 95, 102

Z

OTHER TITLES OF INTEREST FROM HOHM PRESS

10 ESSENTIAL HERBS, Revised Edition
by Lalitha Thomas

Peppermint...Garlic...Ginger...Cayenne...Clove...and five other everyday herbs win the author's vote as the "Top 10" most versatile and effective herbal applications for hundreds of health and beauty needs. *Ten Essential Herbs* offers fascinating stories and easy, step-by-step direction for both beginners and seasoned herbalists. Learn how to use cayenne for headaches, how to make a facial scrub with ginger, how to calm motion sickness and other stomach distress with peppermint. Special sections in each chapter explain the application of these herbs with children and pets too. **Over 25,000 copies in print.**

Paper, 395 pages, $16.95   ISBN: 0-934252-48-3

10 ESSENTIAL FOODS
by Lalitha Thomas

Carrots, broccoli, almonds, grapefruit and six other miracle foods will enhance your health when used regularly and wisely. Lalitha gives in-depth nutritional information plus flamboyant and good-humored stories about these foods, based on her years of health and nutrition counseling. Each chapter contains easy and delicious recipes, tips for feeding kids and helpful hints for managing your food dollar. A bonus section supports the use of 10 Essential Snacks.

Paper, 300 pages, $16.95   ISBN: 0-934252-74-2

TRAVEL HEALTHY
A Guidebook for Health-Conscious Travelers
by Lalitha Thomas

This book will "go" anywhere, whether your itinerary calls for a day trip to your local state park or an odyssey around the world. Lalitha Thomas, author of the highly-acclaimed books *Ten Essential Herbs* and *Ten Essential Foods*, will show you how to prepare a Health-Smart Travel Kit, and how to use it! You'll learn how to apply natural and healthy means to prevent and to remedy dozens of minor emergencies and major inconveniences, like: Indigestion...food poisoning...jet lag...poor water...poor air...colds and flus...toothache...diarrhea...constipation...pesky insects, including bedbugs...sunburn...and more.

Lalitha has traveled extensively, and with children, throughout Mexico, India and Europe. Each chapter contains a section of *Tips for Kids* – simple ways to make their trip more enjoyable and to help them stay healthy on the road, in the air, or on the water.

Paper, 120 pages, $9.95   ISBN: 1-890772-25-9

YOUR BODY CAN TALK: How to Use Simple Muscle Testing to Listen to What Your Body Knows and Needs
by Susan L. Levy, D.C. and Carol Lehr, M.A.

Clear instructions in **simple muscle testing**, together with over 25 simple tests for how to use it for specific problems or disease conditions. Special chapters deal with health problems specific to women (especially PMS and Menopause) and problems specific to men (like stress, heart disease, and prostate difficulties). Contains over 30 diagrams, plus a complete Index and Resource Guide.

Paper, 350 pages, $19.95   ISBN: 0-934252-68-8

To Receive a Full Catalog, or to Order: 800-381-2700
Visit our website at: www.hohmpress.com or use the accompanying Order Form

OTHER TITLES OF INTEREST FROM HOHM PRESS

BEYOND ASPIRIN: *Nature's Challenge To Arthritis, Cancer & Alzheimer's Disease*
by Thomas A. Newmark and Paul Schulick

A reader-friendly guide to one of the most remarkable medical breakthroughs of our times. Research shows that inhibition of the COX-2 enzyme significantly reduces the inflammation that is currently linked with arthritis, colon and other cancers, and Alzheimer's disease. Challenging the conventional pharmaceutical "silver-bullet" approach, this book pleads a convincing case for the safe and effective use of the COX-2-inhibiting herbs, including green tea, rosemary, basil, ginger, turmeric and others.

Paper, 340 pages, $14.95   ISBN: 0-934252-82-3
Cloth, 340 pages, $24.95   ISBN: 1-890772-01-1

GINGER: *Common Spice & Wonder Drug (Third Edition)*
by Paul Schulick

For thousands of years ginger has been one of the world's most favored spices and a major ingredient in Oriental remedies. Yet, ginger's precious healing values are still virtually unknown and ignored in the modern world. This book proposes that ginger is a healing substance beyond the therapeutic scope of any modern drug; a substance with the potential to save billions of dollars and countless lives. Supported by hundreds of scientific studies, this book leads the reader to discover the extraordinary personal and social benefits of using ginger. "A wonderful collection of information. A convincing case." **–Andrew Weil, M.D.**, best-selling author of *Spontaneous Healing*

Paper;176 pages, $9.95   ISBN: 1-890772-07-0

NATURAL HEALING WITH HERBS
by Humbart "Smokey" Santillo, N.D.   Foreword by Robert S. Mendelsohn, M.D.

Dr. Santillo's first book, and Hohm Press's long-standing bestseller, is a classic handbook on herbal and naturopathic treatment. Acclaimed as the most comprehensive work of its kind, *Natural Healing With Herbs* details (in layperson's terms) the properties and uses of 120 of the most common herbs and lists comprehensive therapies for more than 140 common ailments. All in alphabetical order for quick reference.

Paper, 408 pages, $16.95   ISBN: 0-934252-08-4

FOOD ENZYMES — THE MISSING LINK TO RADIANT HEALTH
by Humbart "Smokey" Santillo, N.D.

Santillo's breakthrough book presents the most current research in this field, and encourages simple, straightforward steps for how to make enzyme supplementation a natural addition to a nutrition-conscious lifestyle. Special sections on: longevity and disease; the value of raw food and juicing; detoxification; prevention of allergies and candida; sports and nutrition.

Paper, 108 pages, $7.95   ISBN: 0-934252-40-8 (English)
Paper, 108 pages, $6.95   ISBN: 0-934252-49-1 (Spanish)

Audio version of *Food Enzymes*
2 cassette tapes, 150 minutes, U.S. $17.95   ISBN: 0-934252-29-7

To Receive a Full Catalog, or to Order: 800-381-2700
Visit our website at: www.hohmpress.com or use the accompanying Order Form

OTHER TITLES OF INTEREST FROM HOHM PRESS

THE DETOX MIRACLE SOURCEBOOK
Raw Food and Herbs for Complete Cellular Regeneration
by Robert S. Morse, N.D.

Since 1972, Dr. Morse has directed a health clinic in Florida, successfully helping people cure themselves of cancer, diabetes, M.S., Crohn's disease, along with both brain and nerve damage. His "miracle" approach is fully detailed in this comprehensive book.

Morse's system is to treat the cause of illness, not the symptoms! *The Detox Miracle Sourcebook* is based in Nature. It shows you how to use raw foods and herbs as of the primary means of detoxification, healing, and ultimate regeneration of weak or diseased cells.

Paper, $29.95, 384 pages   ISBN: 1-890772-33-X

THE WILL TO HEALTH
Inertia, Change and Choice
by Robert I. Reynolds, Ph.D., N.D.

The Will to Health is about making the changes that determine our health, and why some people do it, while others apparently don't. But it goes further, pointing to how "the will to live" – which the author calls the "will to health" – can be achieved by working through the natural inertia that normally tends to stop us.

In two-dozen fascinating case studies, Dr. Reynolds, a psychoanalyst and naturopathic physician, introduces us to people with chronic illness who have successfully made a life-saving choice. By clarifying their sense of will or purpose, each patient was able to move beyond their ordinary limits of psychology, belief, or environment.

Paper, 224 pages, $14.95   ISBN: 0-934252-39-9

BUILT TO SURVIVE: HIV Wellness Guide
by Michael Mooney and Nelson Vergel

This first-of-its-kind guide promotes the medical use of anabolic steroids for the HIV(+) population, male and female. An aggressive three-pronged approach (anabolic steroids, nutrition, and exercise) combats the most physically noticeable effect of HIV/AIDS—the loss of lean body mass and weight, known as wasting syndrome.

This book details everything a person with HIV(+) wants to know about anabolic hormones, appetite stimulants, proper diet, cutting edge dietary supplements, and an optimal exercise program to improve health and the potential for long-term survival. Backed with extensive and up-to-the-minute research, this book is both an invaluable resource and a compassionate and brilliant, albeit controversial, handbook to life enhancement.

Paper, 208 pages, $24.95   ISBN: 1-890772-43-7

AFTER SURGERY, ILLNESS OR TRAUMA: 10 Practical Steps to Renewed Energy and Health

by Regina Sara Ryan   Foreword by John W. Travis, M.D.

This book fills the important need of helping us survive and even thrive through our necessary "down-time" in recuperating from surgery, trauma or illness. Learn a wellness approach to recuperation that addresses: how to manage and reduce pain; coping with fear, anger, frustration and other unexpected emotions; keeping inspired for renewed life, during and after recovery; becoming an active participant in your own healing; how to deal with well-meaning visitors and caregivers...and more. Regina Sara Ryan is the co-author, with John W. Travis, M.D. of the classic *Wellness Workbook*, and *Simply Well*.

Paper; 240 pages; $14.95   ISBN: 0-934252-95-5

To Receive a Full Catalog, or to Order: 800-381-2700

Visit our website at: www.hohmpress.com or use the accompanying Order Form

RETAIL ORDER FORM FOR HOHM PRESS

Name _____ Phone (   ) _____

Street Address or P.O. Box _____

City _____ State _____ Zip Code _____

QTY	TITLE	ITEM PRICE	TOTALPRICE
☐	**10 ESSENTIAL HERBS**	**16.95**	
☐	**10 ESSENTIAL FOODS**	**16.95**	
☐	**AFTER SURGERY, ILLNESS OR TRAUMA**	**14.95**	
☐	**BEYOND ASPIRIN (Cloth)**	**24.95**	
☐	**BEYOND ASPIRIN (Paper)**	**14.95**	
☐	**BUILT TO SURVIVE**	**24.95**	
☐	**THE DETOX MIRACLE SOURCEBOOK**	**29.95**	
☐	**FOOD ENZYMES (English)**	**7.95**	
☐	**FOOD ENZYMES (Spanish)**	**6.95**	
☐	**FOOD ENZYMES AUDIO TAPES**	**17.95**	
☐	**GINGER**	**9.95**	
☐	**NATURAL HEALING WITH HERBS**	**16.95**	
☐	**TRAVEL HEALTHY**	**9.95**	
☐	**THE WILL TO HEALTH**	**14.95**	
☐	**YOUR BODY CAN TALK**	**19.95**	

SUBTOTAL:

SHIPPING:
(see right)

TOTAL:

SURFACE SHIPPING CHARGES:
1st book or tape item ....$5.00   Each additional item .....add $1.00

SHIP MY ORDER:
- ☐ Surface U.S. Mail–Priority   ☐ Fex-Ex Ground (Mail + $3.00)
- ☐ 2nd Day Air (Mail + $5.00)   ☐ Next Day Air (Mail + $15.00)

METHOD OF PAYMENT:
- ☐ Check or M.O.   Payable to Hohm Press, P.O. Box 2501, Prescott, AZ 86302
- ☐ Call 1-800-381-2700 to place your credit card order
- ☐ Or call 1-928-717-1779 to fax your credit card order
- ☐ Information for Visa/MasterCard/American Express order only:

Card#_____-_____-_____-_____ Expiration Date: _____

To Receive a Full Catalog, or to Order: 800-381-2700
Visit our website at: www.hohmpress.com or use the accompanying Order Form

About the Authors

Michael Mooney is a journalist and nutritional researcher and advocate for holistic therapies in the treatment of HIV. He is the director of research and communication for PoWeR (Program for Wellness Restoration). He has published a regular newsletter promoting their work, and maintained their comprehensive website: www.medibolics.com. Michael has given hundreds of lectures on this subject, been interviewed by *Sports Illustrated*, quoted on *Good Morning America*, and has published articles in various publications in the U.S. and worldwide, including: *European AIDS Treatment News*, *Musclemag*, *Ironman* and *Muscle Media*. He lives in Los Angeles.

Nelson Vergel, chemical engineer, founder of Program for Wellness Restoration, and the Body Wellness Center/Houston, has been HIV(+) since 1983. He experimented with the principles set forth in *Built to Survive* and is living proof of their effectiveness. Nelson has given hundreds of lectures since 1994 throughout the United States, in Europe, and in South America, and is a leading treatment advocate in the U.S. "The time has come to treat HIV comprehensively with not only anti-retrovirals, but also with life-enhancing complementary therapies...Minimizing the side effects of drug therapies is key to living better and longer. We hope we can make it easier to conquer many of them with our book," says Vergel. He lives in Houston, Texas.

To contact Michael or Nelson, or to review updates of *Built to Survive* information, visit www.medibolics.com and www.facialwasting.org

* * *

All of the authors' net proceeds from the sale of *Built to Survive* will fund nonprofit organizations focusing on HIV wellness.